THE
SURGERY
HANDBOOK

A GUIDE TO UNDERSTANDING
YOUR OPERATION

PAUL RUGGIERI, M.D.

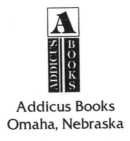

Addicus Books
Omaha, Nebraska

An Addicus Nonfiction Book

ISBN 1-886039-38-0

Cover design by Robert Aulicino
Typography by Linda Dageforde

This book is not intended to serve as a substitute for a physician, nor does the author intend to give medical advice contrary to that of an attending physician.

Library of Congress Cataloging-in-Publication Data
Ruggieri, Paul, 1959-
    The surgery handbook : a guide to understanding your operation / Paul Ruggieri.
        p. cm.
Includes bibliographical references (p.) and index.
    ISBN 1-886039-38-0 (alk. paper)
    1. Surgery—Popular works. I. Title.
    RD31.3.R845 2000
    617—c21

                                                                99-050492

                        Addicus Books, Inc.
                          P.O. Box 45327
                       Omaha, Nebraska 68145
                  Web site: http://www.AddicusBooks.com

              Printed in the United States of America
                    10 9 8 7 6 5 4 3 2 1

To Rick,
I hope you never need This book.
However if you ever need surgery
just call me

To my parents, John and Irene,
for their unconditional support of
my dream to become a surgeon.

Contents

Acknowledgments

I could not have completed this book without the support of many special people. First and foremost, I thank my patients for the many lessons they have taught me. All have been instrumental in helping me assemble the contents of this book. I also thank Rod Colvin of Addicus Books and his staff for their belief in this project, as well as editor Anne Greenberg for her tireless efforts. I appreciate, too, the help of John Bartimole. I thank Larry Connors for his inspiration in converting this book from an idea to the written word. I thank Robert Wiltshire for his help with the information about anesthesia.

I extend sincere thanks to the staff at Middle Tennessee Surgical Associates in Columbia, Tennessee. Clare Keller and her staff have been an extended family to me. I also thank Dr. Cary Pulliam and Dr. Mark Shelton, two outstanding surgeons, for giving me opportunities and friendship.

Finally, I acknowledge the staff and surgeons of Truesdale Surgical Associates in Massachusetts. Dr. Jerry Monchik, Dr. Dan Eardley, and Dr. Robert Sandfort have all been great in helping me return home.

Introduction

Perhaps you've stood at the bedside of friends and relatives who have undergone surgery. You were glad to be there, offering them your full support. But now, *you're* about to become the patient, a prospect you may find a bit frightening. Rest assured, your reaction is normal. Just mention *surgery*, and even the strongest soul may feel weak in the knees. No one looks forward to surgery.

Still, learn all you can about your operation and recovery. It is one of the most helpful things you can do. You can reduce anxiety and fear of the unknown by gathering information. Knowledge is power. That is why I decided to write this book. As a general surgeon, I spend hours answering my patients' questions about every aspect of surgery and hospitalization. I believe this interaction is essential to their well-being. My patients are much better prepared to undergo surgery because they know what they are facing.

Because every individual is different, it is impossible to offer specifics about every surgical procedure. Still, I am confident that this book will help you understand the basics of surgery. I chose surgery as a profession because I wished to see immediately the results of my work helping people. In this same spirit, I trust that you will benefit from this book.

Chapter 1

So You Need Surgery

You've just learned that you need surgery. Perhaps you've suspected it for some time. Or, perhaps your diagnosis came as a complete surprise. Whatever your situation, the days or weeks ahead may take you down a path you may not have traveled before. It may be emotionally unsettling.

Why is it so difficult to accept the need for surgery? Most of us fear losing control of our lives. If we're not in control, we fear something could go wrong. We also fear that we may die. This is especially true when a diagnosis involves a life-threatening illness like cancer or heart disease and surgery needs to be performed immediately.

Your fear may also stem from the negative experience of a relative who had a similar operation. You may fear pain after the operation. You may be frightened because you don't know if your job will be waiting for you when you are able to go back to work. These are all legitimate fears. It is normal to experience them.

Alleviating Anxiety

It may take a while for you to accept the need for surgery. If the upcoming operation is creating a lot of anxiety for you, there are several ways to reduce it.

Education

Often, simply knowing the facts will quell your anxiety. There is no shortage of information available today through libraries and the Internet. This book will answer a number of your questions and guide you to a variety of resources. You might also find it helpful to visit someone who has had the same surgery and done well. Finally, you'll also feel better knowing that you're in the hands of a competent surgeon.

Patients today have many more options when having surgery. Part of my job is making them aware of these options so an informed decision can be made by all.

Cary, 45, M.D.
Surgeon

Exercise

Unless you've received instructions to the contrary, you may exercise right up to the time you enter the hospital. According to scientific studies, physical exercise is good for both the body and the mind. In a study done at the University of Wisconsin in 1978, exercise was shown to be effective in treating depression and anxiety. In the study, patients who received only therapy for depression, did not recover as fast as those who also exercised. Exercise also promotes better sleep.

Medication

If your anxiety persists, relief is available in the form of antianxiety medications. Although such drugs may not be recommended just days before an operation, other medications may help bring your anxiety under control. Talk to your primary care physician about your options if your anxiety persists.

Meditation

Meditation and relaxation exercises may also lessen your stress level. Practice relaxing your body in a quiet place free of disruptions. Perhaps you find music relaxing. Many people recommend using an audiotape that leads you through exercises in which you typically practice rhythmic breathing and concentrate on relaxing one part of your body at a time. Others find that visualization, in which you create a picture of corrective action taking place, helps to drain tension away.

Including Your Family and Friends

Your diagnosis will certainly affect others in your life. Family and friends will most likely want to rally around you with love and support. While some people like to "go it alone," you will probably find it most helpful to rely on a network of support. Remember, this is a stressful time for you. Even if you are used to being self-sufficient, this is a good time to let others help you. Support from family and friends will help you mentally as well as physically. They can take some of the burden of handling daily activities off your shoulders so that you can focus on getting well.

> *It took several days for it to sink in that I had cancer and needed further surgery. Once I became determined to beat it, I did some research and listed many questions about my disease and surgery.*
>
> *Martha, 55*
> *Patient*

Chapter 2

Choosing a Surgeon

You may not need to select a surgeon to perform your operation. It is quite common for a primary care physician to recommend a qualified surgeon, and you may be comfortable with this. Or you may already know of a surgeon whom you'd prefer. However, if you need to find a surgeon, many sources of information are available to help with your selection.

For those with access to the Internet, a wealth of information is available online. Many states have web sites on the Internet listing all the practicing surgeons, their areas of expertise, and biographical data. There are also various web sites devoted to health care that allow you to search for hospitals, physicians, and surgeons based on specialty and location. For example, at healthgrades.com, you may get tips on choosing a physician and ask for listings of surgeons and physicians in any state.

Consider nearby prominent universities, medical schools, and well-known clinics. They often have national reputations for their expertise in specific areas, like cancer, heart surgery, and sports medicine. Because these centers do a great deal of research and often develop new medical procedures, their staffs include highly qualified professionals.

Other sources include friends and relatives, state medical societies, the yellow pages, insurance companies, and patient-services departments of hospitals.

Checking a Surgeon's Credentials

When you have a surgeon in mind or when one has been recommended, it is wise to check both his/her credentials as well as experience in the operating room.

It may also be helpful to understand how surgeons are educated and trained.

Experience in the Operating Room

It's important to know how much practical experience the surgeon has. Ask how many times the surgeon has performed operations like the one you're having. You'll want a surgeon with considerable experience. Of course, the term *experience* means different things to different people. It's difficult to pinpoint the exact number of operations a surgeon should have done to be considered experienced. You might ask how many of these operations the surgeon does a month, a year.

I knew nothing about my surgeon except that he was recommended by my family physician. I had no idea I needed a specialist. Luckily, everything worked out and the surgeon was great. If I had to do it over again I would ask more questions.

Cathy, 47
Patient

If the surgeon does only a few per year, he/she may lack experience. Also ask the surgeon how he/she has handled complications with this type of surgery in the operating room.

Complaints or Sanctions

It's also important to know whether a surgeon has had any complaints or sanctions lodged against him/her. This may be a bit difficult for you to ask directly. However, every state has a government agency that oversees its physicians, a board or department of medical examiners. This agency not only oversees the licensing of physicians but also investigates and rules on complaints against doctors. You have the right to know if a surgeon is under scrutiny by this agency for any reason. Many states allow you to contact their agency online and can provide you with information regarding any complaints.

Training/Medical School

After finishing four years of college, medical students must complete another four years of medical school. The first half of medical school is devoted to classroom and laboratory work. The last two years involve patient care in hospital settings. After these eight years, students earn their doctor of medicine (M.D.) degree.

Additional Training for Surgery

As graduates of medical school, new doctors lack the skills and experience to perform surgery. They all must undertake additional hands-on training in whatever specialty they choose. This additional training, called a *residency*, may last from five to eight years. Most surgical residencies are based at university teaching hospitals; however, some integrate larger community hospitals as well. During this period, surgical residents care for patients and perform surgery under the direct supervision of board-certified, fully trained surgeons. When their training is finished, the surgeons are given a diploma by the institution certifying their residency. They are now considered qualified to practice surgery on their own.

Board Certification

Once in practice, new surgeons are given five years in which to pass a rigorous written and oral examination to become board-certified by the body governing their specialty, in many cases the American Board of Surgery. This certification is the final stamp of approval given to all surgeons in practice. Every surgeon should be able to attain board certification during the first five years of practice, yet about one-third of U.S. surgeons are not board-certified in any specialty. Patients may have legitimate concerns about an uncertified surgeon's ability to perform surgery safely.

Fellowship

Another level of training for some surgical specialties is a *fellowship*. Not all surgeons are or need to be fellowship trained. Most surgeons learn what they need to know during a comprehensive five- or six-year surgical residency. But if you are facing a complex blood-vessel operation, it is comforting to know that your surgeon has spent one to two additional years operating only on blood vessels.

Patients place a lot of blind trust in the system when being referred to a surgeon. Most patients have no idea whether their surgeon is board certified or even a specialist. I try to reassure them by explaining who I am and what I do.

Steve, 38, M.D.
Cancer Surgeon

Do I Need a Second Opinion?

If you believe your diagnosis is accurate, you probably won't need to seek another physician's opinion. On the other hand, the second opinion of another medical doctor or surgeon may provide you with peace of mind that the original diagnosis is correct. A second opinion is a good idea if (1) the first physician is not certain of the diagnosis because your tests are inconclusive or (2) if a life-threatening disease, such as severe heart disease or cancer, has been diagnosed. Keep in mind that most doctors are not offended by your seeking another opinion. In fact, many doctors welcome it. Doctors are accustomed to their patients seeking another opinion.

I have developed strong relationships with several surgeons in the community and trust in their judgment and skills. When I refer a patient to a particular surgeon, I feel confident that patient will get the best of care.
Joseph, 44, M.D.
Internist

Before getting a second opinion, you may want to ask the second physician about referring to your first set of test results, including X-rays and other films. Your insurance company may not pay for duplicate tests. It's a good idea to call your insurance company first to find out if they will cover the expense of getting a second opinion.

With an HMO Do I Still Have a Choice?

There is no single right answer to this question because there are so many different insurance plans available. There are even differences in plans within a single state, depending on which options people choose when they enroll. To find out whether you may choose your surgeon, check with your insurance company.

Almost every health maintenance organization (HMO) and preferred provider organization (PPO) offers some flexibility in choosing a physician. You probably selected your primary care physician from a list of doctors, and you may be able to choose from a list of surgeons as well.

May I Choose My Hospital?

Again, the answer will have to come from your insurance company. Your insurance plan may cover you only if you go to a hospital on the plan (except in emergencies). Additionally, doctors usually cannot send a patient to any hospital; they must have admitting privileges at that hospital. If needed, doctors usually can apply for temporary admitting privileges, but they will not be as familiar with the hospital.

There is a great deal of difference among hospitals. The right hospital for you may also vary, depending on the type of surgery and care you need. For example, if you're going in for a minor biopsy, a local community hospital should be sufficient. But if you're facing a complex procedure, you'll need to be at a larger hospital where a full range of health care specialists will be available. Many hospitals affiliated with teaching universities are set up to handle difficult cases. Accordingly, such hospitals usually have good reputations.

If you have any concerns about the hospital you'll be visiting, you may first check it out through the Joint Commission for Accreditation of health care Organizations (JCAHO). Membership in this organization indicates that the facility has voluntarily met established standards regarding delivery of care and services.

Chapter 3

Learning about Your Operation

You probably have many questions about your surgery and recovery. You'll fare better emotionally and physically if you have a clear understanding of what your operation will entail. Therefore, don't hesitate to ask questions and re-ask them if you are not clearly understanding an answer. The surgeon and his/her staff will be your best source of information. Don't feel intimidated or think the surgeon will be offended by your questions. You and your loved ones have a right to know all about your operation.

Asking Questions of Your Physician

Below is a list of questions that you may wish to ask your surgeon and his/her staff. Carry the list with you. It may be very helpful to jot down answers to your questions. Better yet, ask a friend or relative to take notes for you. It's easy to misunderstand an answer, especially if you're a bit nervous.

In General

- What is my specific physical problem? What organ, system, or body part is involved?
- What does this organ/system/body part do?
- What is causing the problem I now have?
- Will surgery cure the problem?
- Are there alternative treatments that don't involve surgery? How do they compare with surgery? Are they as effective? Safe?
- What would happen if I don't have surgery?

The Procedure

- On which part of my body will you perform the operation?
- How long will the incision be?
- Approximately how long will the surgery take?
- Do you consider this major surgery?
- How many of these surgeries do you perform in a year?
- Is it a standard procedure or is it experimental?

Postoperative Concerns

- Where will I be when I wake up?
- Will I be in pain upon awakening? If so, how long will it last?
- When I wake up, will I have any tubes in my body? If so, for how long?
- How long will I be in the recovery room?

Possible Complications

- What can go wrong with this type of surgery?
- How often do these complications occur?
- Am I likely to have complications?

- What happens if one of these complications does occur? How will it be treated? Could it cause permanent damage?
- Have any of your patients experienced these complications?

Post-Surgical Care

- After the operation, will I go to a regular room or to a special unit?
- How long before I may go home?
- May I have visitors in the hospital and at home?
- Will I be on a restricted diet in the hospital or at home?
- Will I receive any sort of therapy in the hospital?
- Will I receive any medication while in the hospital?
- Do the nurses know to give me the medications that I already take?
- Will I be able to drive myself home from the hospital, or should someone take me?
- Will I need any specialized care or help when I go home?
- Do I have limits physically?
- At home, will I need any medical equipment (crutches, portable toilet, ventilator)? If so, how may I get this equipment?
- Should I call your office if I'm having a problem?

Recovery

- When should I see you in your office after surgery?
- When can I go back to work? Drive? Exercise? Have sex? Work out?
- Do I need physical therapy?

You will have other questions of your own to ask your surgeon. Don't hesitate. Communication between you and your surgeon is extremely important from the moment you meet until the time you leave your surgeon's care. Ask, ask, ask questions!

No matter how thorough your surgeon staff, always ask for written information about your condition and your surgery. They may have instructions, brochures, books, or even videos that show your procedure and recovery. Still others may provide you with a CD-ROM for your computer that combines audio and video clips with written material about your operation. You may review these materials over and over again to help you feel more comfortable about your surgery.

Online Research

If you have access to the Internet, you also may conduct research about your condition. Using a word or phrase, your computer may search through general databases and web sites around the world. Be forewarned that you may come across a web site that sounds authentic but is created by someone who has no credentials to write a medical page. That's why it's a good idea to stay with sites from established organizations or facilities that you recognize.

Most patients are afraid to ask questions. They think I will be offended by being asked if I have done this operation before. This is so untrue. Most surgeons realize the anxiety associated with surgery and invite questions.

Mark, 40
Vascular Surgeon

When doctors do research online, they frequently use a database called MEDLINE, which is compiled by the U.S. National Medical Library (NLM), the world's largest medical library. NLM is part of the National Institutes of Health and may be reached at http://www.nlm.nih.gov. You will find other databases there as well. MEDLINE contains references from approximately 3,900 international medical journals from the year 1966 to the present. Note: these articles are written for medical professionals, so they may be difficult to understand.

You will likely find the NLM's companion site, MEDLINEplus, more reader friendly. It may also be reached at http://www.nlm.nih.gov. It was developed for the general public when the NLM discovered that one-third of nearly 200 million MEDLINE searches were being done by consumers. MEDLINEplus is an up-to-date collection of consumer health care information. It is free for consumers, health care professionals, and scientists.

For most patients and families, the anxiety of having an operation is mostly not knowing what will happen next. The day of the surgery, I spend as much time as possible trying to make sure that anxieties are relieved.

Paul, 39, M.D.
Surgeon

Organizations

Organizations dedicated to educating people about specific conditions or problems are excellent resources. Some well-known examples are the American Heart Association, American Diabetes Association, Muscular Dystrophy Association, and the American Cancer Society (see Resources). Many major organizations have Internet sites that offer a great deal of information. They also have local and national offices that will mail printed materials. Several have telephone help lines you may call with your questions.

Chapter 4

Pain Management

Another important issue you'll want to discuss with your surgeon is pain control. None of us like the thought of experiencing pain. In fact, post-operative pain may be one of our biggest fears about having surgery. And unfortunately, such fear is not unfounded. According to the federal government's Agency for Health Care Policy and Research, nearly fifty percent of all post-surgical pain is under treated. In this chapter, we'll examine both why post-surgical pain is so often inadequately treated, and what you can do to ensure that you do not suffer undue pain after your operation.

Barriers to Effective Pain Management

It's difficult to believe, in this age of modern medicine, that half the 23 million patients who undergo surgery experience moderate to severe pain after their operations. How could this be, you ask? There is not a single answer to the question; rather the barriers to effective pain management are created by a combination of problems involving patients, health care professionals, and health care institutions.

Problems Related to Patients
- Reluctance to report pain
- Concern about distracting physicians from treatment of underlying disease
- Fear that pain means the disease is worse
- Concern about being a "good" patient
- Reluctance to take pain medications
- Fear of addiction or of being thought of as an addict
- Worries about unmanageable side effects of pain medications
- Concern about becoming tolerant of pain medications

Problems Related to Health Care Professionals
- Poor assessment of pain
- Inadequate knowledge of pain management
- Concern about regulation of controlled substances
- Fear of patient addiction
- Concern about side affects of analgesics
- Concern about patients becoming tolerant of analgesics

Problems Related to the Health Care System
- Inadequate reimbursement
- Restrictive regulation of controlled substances
- Problems of availability of treatment or access to treatment
- Low priority given to pain treatment for cancer

Clearly, fear of addiction is the largest, single barrier to pain control. Addiction refers to the continued self-administration of a substance in spite of social disapproval or negative consequences in one's life. However, research shows that taking pain medication after surgery to manage legitimate pain does not lead to addiction. Still, temporary physical dependence on a narcotic is often confused with addiction. With the temporary dependence, your cells can become accustomed to a drug taken over a period of time, and you would feel the effects of withdrawal if the drug were stopped abruptly. Accordingly, when it is time to stop the drug, your physician will gradually taper down the dosages. This short-term cellular dependence is not to be compared with the destructive, drug-seeking behaviors of addiction.

Planning for Your Pain Control

Studies show that patients armed with knowledge of pain management report less pain, use less medication, and leave the hospital earlier than those who have no idea what to expect in the area of pain after surgery. Education and planning is the key to ensuring that your pain is adequately treated. As an informed patient, you can develop a Pain Control Plan, in which you and your doctor map out a plan for how your pain will be alleviated. The following guidelines will be helpful in formulating a plan.

- What is your physician's approach to pain control?
- Tell your doctors and nurses about your concerns and methods that have worked well for you in the past.
- Ask if the hospital has a pain service provided by an anesthesiologist or physician who specializes in pain management. This service may be called upon should your pain not be under control.
- Assign your pain a number value to help doctors and nurses know how well your treatment is working. Report your pain on a scale of 0 to 10. Set a goal, such as having no pain worse than 2 on the scale.

- Take pain-relief drugs as soon as the pain starts. This is a key step in proper pain control.
- If your pain will likely worsen when you start walking or moving, take the pain medication first. It's harder to ease pain once it has started.
- Draft a plan for treating your pain after you leave the hospital.

Sample Pain Control Plan

Pain control plan for _____

your name

Before surgery, I will take _____.

name of medication

How will I use the medication? _____

After surgery, my pain will be controlled with _____ in the hospital.

name of medication

This medication will be given to me

_____ as pill _____ by IV _____ as a shot _____ through a tube in my back.

I will receive the medication
_____ at certain times
_____ every _____ hours for _____ days
_____ around the clock
_____ when I call the nurse

I will also use these non-drug pain-control methods in the hospital and at home: _____

_____ (list methods)

At home, I will take _____

name of medication

From the National Institutes for Health

Medications & Delivery Methods

With a plan for pain control in place, let's examine the methods used for pain management. The drugs most used to relieve pain are *analgesics*. The methods through which they can be given include: pill, injection, *intravenous line (IV)*, or suppository. Analgesics are usually divided into two categories: *opioids* and *non-opioids*.

Opioids

These include narcotics such as morphine, demerol, codeine, and similar drugs. Narcotics actually work in the brain, not only blocking pain signals but also producing a sedative effect. They are highly effective against postoperative pain. It is important, too, to understand their possible side effects. Often your physician can give you additional medications to relieve any unpleasant side effects.

Possible Side Effects
- nausea
- itching
- constipation
- bladder not emptying regularly

Non-opioids

These include aspirin, acetaminophen, ibuprofen, and other nonsteroidal, anti-inflammatory drugs. These work to check pain at its source. However, they are much slower to act than opioids. These nonnarcotic analgesics are best for mild pain.

Possible Side Effects
- gastric irritation
- interference with blood clotting

Patient-Controlled Analgesia (PCA)

Patient-controlled analgesia (PCA) allows a patient to administer his/her own continuous pain relief. An intravenous line is attached to a pump. The patient presses a button to administer a dose of an analgesic when needed. The pump may be programmed to limit how much of the drug may be given in a specified time period. The PCA is widely used in the United States because it works well and has a good safety record. Patients often use less medication than with the old injection method. It's important to learn how to use the unit properly before surgery.

Don't wait until you're in pain to think about a pain control plan. Go into your surgery with a plan.
Betty F., R.N., Ph.D. Pain Research Scientist

For patients who had epidural or spinal anesthesia, PCA is readily available since a small thin tube, inserted in the back for the anesthesia, can be left in place. The tube can be attached to the pump so that the painkilling medication may be administered directly. However, one side effect of this method is weakness in the legs. The patient needs to stay in bed if it is to be used.

In the past, before PCA was available, a narcotic was administered only when a patient asked for it, only *after* he/she began to feel pain. The narcotic was usually given by injection only in four-hour intervals. Unfortunately, for many patients the effect wore off before another shot was allowed. This left the patient in quite a bit of pain during that four-hour time frame, despite receiving other pain killers.

Injecting the Incision

Another method for immediate pain relief is to inject an anesthetic near or into the incision. Such local anesthetics are effective for severe pain. With this approach, there is no drowsiness, constipation or problem with breathing. An injection may reduce the need for opioids.

Alternative Solutions

Other methods that do not involve medications may be used to relieve pain. They may not work as well on intense pain, but they may assist with moderate pain and may even reinforce the pain-relieving effects of drugs.

I try to let patients know how they will feel immediately after waking up from their anesthesia. I also reassure them that we have many ways of making them comfortable and pain free.

> *Ralph, 53, M.D.*
> *Anesthesiologist*

TENS Unit

Your surgeon may prescribe a *transcutaneous electrical nerve stimulation (TENS)* unit. This unit uses low-level electrical stimulation to block the pain impulses around your incision. It is about the size of a pager and attaches to your body by electrodes. Many patients find the unit quite helpful, although it loses effectiveness as the nerves adapt to it. There are few risks associated with TENS, although the electrodes may irritate your skin.

Cold Packs

Applied directly, cold packs may bring relief by temporarily numbing the painful area.

Relaxation and Massage

Some patients find meditation and relaxation helpful. Try simple abdominal breathing exercises and relaxing your jaw or more complex meditation techniques. You need no equipment and may use these techniques any time. Tense muscles in other parts of your body may be intensifying pain. If so, massage may help bring some measure of comfort. Massage should be used with the approval of your surgeon to make sure it does not affect the incision.

The intense pain you originally felt after surgery normally fades in two or three days by itself. If it doesn't, then you may be experiencing a complication. However, if all goes well, your pain medication will be adjusted to lower doses as you continue to recover and move toward your release from the hospital.

Chapter 5

Risk Factors

With surgery, everyone hopes for the best possible results. Still, it is often difficult to predict the outcome. Many surgeries are rather predictable, while others are less certain. The outcome may be influenced by risk factors present at the time of your operation. Every surgery carries with it a certain amount of risk. Generally, the more complex the surgery, the higher the risk that something could go wrong. For example, the risk involved in open-heart surgery is certainly greater than that for carpal tunnel syndrome. Your health care team carefully considers risk factors that may impact your surgery and recovery.

Age

As you age, your risk of developing diseases increases. For instance, one in ten women in the United States between the ages of 45 and 64 has heart disease, but this number jumps to one in four for women 65 and older. There are many reasons. Lower estrogen levels due to menopause reduce certain protections to the heart. The level of cholesterol in the blood increases as women age. Higher blood pressure, reduced physical activity, increased weight, and diabetes are also common factors. Aging is a natural occurrence for all of us, affecting our strength and stamina.

Weight

The more weight you carry, the higher your risk not only of surgical complications but also of numerous other conditions that are, in themselves, risk factors for surgery. These include coronary heart disease, stroke, high blood pressure, high cholesterol, and diabetes.

My biggest fear going into my back surgery was fearing the operation would not correct the terrible pain I had been experiencing. I did have confidence in the surgical team and ultimately had a very good result.

Robert, 38
Patient

Being overweight means your body has to work harder. For example, your heart must pump blood into additional tissue created by extra fat. Further, your heart may have to expend more effort to push blood through vessels that may be clogged with plaque from a higher cholesterol level brought on by the increased weight. If you are overweight, it is likely that you are also physically inactive. This means your muscles are also probably out of shape and will have to work harder still to help you recover.

Smoking

Smoking is risk factor for many diseases. These, in turn, may heighten your risk during surgery. Smoking increases your risk of stroke, heart attack, coronary heart disease, chronic obstructive lung diseases, and cancer. Smoking may bring even greater health risks when combined with other illnesses. For example, the cardiovascular risks of smoking and diabetes combined are fourteen times those of either factor alone. If you smoke, your lungs do not exchange oxygen as easily as those of nonsmokers, which may affect how your body responds to general anesthesia.

Alcohol Abuse

Alcohol abuse may increase blood pressure and contribute to heart disease, stroke, and liver disease. Alcohol also contains no nutrients—only calories—and may lead to weight gain.

Other Medical Conditions

Other medical conditions may also increase your surgical risk. Almost without exception, these conditions require multiple medications, creating the potential for dangerous interactions among the drugs themselves, with anesthesia, and/or with any other drugs prescribed for surgery. These factors increase the risk of complications.

Before and after my breast cancer surgery, I had a ton of questions. My surgeon sat down with me for as long as it took to ease my anxieties. When I left his office I felt very satisfied and determined about beating breast cancer.

Edith, 45
Nurse and Patient

Hypertension

High blood pressure, or hypertension, occurs when the pressure against artery walls is elevated as blood passes through. The added pressure may weaken arteries. Subsequently, arteries may burst or cause blood clots, which in turn may lead to stroke or heart failure.

Diabetes

Diabetics typically suffer hypertension, which makes the heart work harder. Hypertension in turn increases their risk of stroke or heart attack during surgery. In addition, diabetes often leads to damage to other organs, such as the kidneys, which also increases risk. Diabetics, overall, do not heal well and are at increased risk of postoperative complications like bedsores.

Heart disease

If the heart is already weakened by disease, the added strain of surgery may increase the chances of heart attack or stroke.

High cholesterol

Increased amounts of cholesterol and fat, adhering to the walls of arteries, decrease blood flow. This in turn increases the risk of developing coronary heart disease.

Arthritis

People living with the pain of arthritis often use anti-inflammatory or analgesic medications. These drugs may lead to stomach and ulcer problems, which in turn may increase gastric bleeding. Many such drugs also thin the blood, which only heightens the risk of excessive bleeding during surgery.

As you'll note, many risks are based on lifestyle. Other factors—positive or negative—are beyond one's control. For example, your body may naturally heal quickly. Or, the width of your blood vessels might make you a good candidate for heart-bypass surgery. You may have strong, healthy bones, which may bring swift recovery from surgery to repair a broken ankle. A number of such factors may influence your recovery.

Chapter 6

Types of Surgery

It is estimated between 23 and 25 million surgeries are performed annually in the United States. Having surgery means anything from fifteen minutes in an ophthalmologist's office to remove a cyst from an eyelid to hours in an operating room undergoing a liver transplant. Every day, tens of thousands of operations are performed. In general, these fall into three basic categories: major, minor, and the newer minimally invasive surgeries.

Minor Surgery

Minor surgery involves only small incisions and may require little recovery time, let alone time in the hospital. Minor surgery includes procedures such as:

- biopsies
- vasectomy
- removal of cysts and warts
- treatment of localized infections
- many ear surgeries
- cataract removal
- tubal ligation
- correction of lazy eye
- setting fractures
- small skin grafts

Major Surgery

The traditional view most of us have of an operation is *major surgery*. We think in terms of incisions, hospital stays, and recuperation. Indeed, this is often the case with major surgery, also known as *invasive* or *open surgery*. The body is opened with an incision, usually several inches long, allowing surgeons to place their hands inside the body cavity to work. Invasive surgery causes more postoperative pain, and the recovery period is longer. Major surgery includes procedures such as:

- organ transplants
- heart surgery (coronary-artery bypass, valve replacement)
- removal of cancerous tumors
- brain surgery (aneurysms, tumors)
- abdominal or gastrointestinal surgery (stomach, colon)
- joint replacement (hip, knee, shoulder)
- back and neck surgery
- abdominal aortic aneurysm repairs
- carotid-artery surgery
- chest and lung surgery
- major facial reconstructive surgery
- gynecologic surgery (removal of uterus, ovaries)
- kidney removal
- bladder and prostate-gland surgery
- spleen removal

Minimally Invasive Surgery

Thanks to modern medicine, *minimally invasive surgery* has become common practice. As the name suggests, it is less invasive to the body. Incisions are small. Surgeons do not place their hands inside the body cavity. Such operations are far less traumatic to the body, so patients recover more quickly.

You may have heard of a minimally invasive technique called *laparoscopic surgery*. It was originally introduced in the early 1970s for gynecologic operations but has since been applied to other procedures. It is also referred to as *keyhole* or *pinhole surgery* because of the small incisions made. For instance, a surgeon may make a quarter-inch incision in a patient's navel, inserting into the abdominal cavity a *laparoscope*, a narrow wand containing a tiny video camera. Working with other tools also inserted through small incisions, the surgeon may then remove a diseased appendix, for example. The video camera acts as the surgeon's eyes, projecting the image onto a television screen. The picture is magnified twenty times, allowing the surgeon to see minute details that otherwise might be missed with the naked eye. Laparoscopic surgeries include procedures such as:

I surprised my surgeon by asking how many of these laparoscopic procedures he had performed. I just wanted to make sure I wasn't the first. He was honest and receptive with his answers and made me feel confident in his abilities.

Martha, 55
Patient

- gallbladder removal
- appendix removal
- hernia repair
- uterus and ovary removal
- colon removal
- partial lung removal
- spleen removal
- surgery for chronic heartburn or reflux disease (GERD)

With laparoscopic surgery incisions are smaller, the patient suffers less postoperative pain, hospital stays are shorter, and recovery is quicker.

Common Operations

Listed below are some of the most common operations. Also shown are the estimated times to perform and recover from surgery. Please note: since recovery varies among individuals, these times are only approximations. The time to perform operations may also vary in length, depending on circumstances.

General Surgery
- gallbladder removal (*cholecystectomy*)
- hernia repair
- appendix removal (*appendectomy*)
- breast biopsies and breast removal for cancer
- thyroid gland removal (*thyroidectomy*)
- stomach surgery
- intestinal surgery
- *Length of Operation:* 15 minutes for outpatient breast biopsy to several hours for pancreas removal.
- *Recovery Time:* 1-8 weeks

Cardiothoracic Surgery
- coronary-artery bypass graft surgery (CABG)
- heart valve replacement
- removal of a portion of a lung, mainly performed for cancer (*lobectomy*)
- removal of the esophagus, mainly performed for cancer (*esophagectomy*)

- *Length of Operation*: 2-8 hours
- *Recovery Time*: 4-8 weeks

Colorectal Surgery

- removal of any portion of the colon, mainly for cancer, growths, or diverticular disease (*colectomy*)
- gallbladder removal (*cholecystectomy*)
- removal of hemorrhoids (*hemorrhoidectomy*)
- internally examine the colon with a fiber-optic scope (*colonoscopy*)
- internally examine the stomach with a fiber-optic scope (*endoscopy*)
- *Length of Operation:* 30 minutes for an outpatient hemorrhoidectomy to 3 hours to remove part of the colon.
- *Recovery Time:* 1-8 weeks

Ear, Nose, and Throat (ENT) Surgery (Otolaryngology)

- ear-tube placement in children for recurrent infections
- sinus surgery for diseased sinuses
- surgery for cancer of the mouth, salivary glands, throat, and larynx
- thyroid gland removal (*thyroidectomy*)
- cosmetic facial surgery
- *Length of Operation:* 1-2 hours for outpatient ENT procedures. Operations for cancer of the head and neck are longer and more complex.
- *Recovery Time:* 1-8 weeks

Gynecologic Surgery

- removal of the uterus (*hysterectomy*)

- clipping the fallopian tubes to prevent reproduction (*tubal ligation*)
- removal of fallopian tubes and ovaries (*salpingo-oophorectomy*)
- examination of the reproductive organs with a fiber-optic scope (*laparoscopy*)
- opening the uterus to allow the birth of a baby (*cesarean section*)
- *Length of Operation:* 1-3 hours
- *Recovery Time:* 2-4 weeks

Neurosurgery

- removal of brain tumors, blood clots
- repairing a brain aneurysm (*craniotomy*)
- removal of a piece of bone from the spinal column, relieving pressure on nerves (*laminectomy*)
- full or partial removal of a disc in the spinal column to release pressure on nerves (*disc decompression*)
- removal of plaque blocking arteries in the neck (*carotid endarterectomy*)
- *Length of Operation:* 1-2 hours for a disc decompression or up to 6-10 hours to remove a complex brain tumor.
- *Recovery Time:* 2-8 weeks

Oncologic Surgery

- Surgery for cancer in any part of the body including removal of tumors in the breast, thyroid, intestines, liver, pancreas, stomach, and brain.
- *Length of Operation:* 2-6 hours
- *Recovery Time:* 2-8 weeks

Orthopedic Surgery

- total joint replacement (commonly the hip among the elderly)
- rebuilding a damaged joint (joint reconstruction)
- arthroscopic joint surgery (joint repair, most commonly the knee)
- open reduction and internal fixation, or ORIF (placing pins, metal rods, and other devices around broken bones to speed healing)
- removal of bone from the spinal column to remove pressure on nerves *(lumbar laminectomy)*
- *Length of Operation:* 30 minutes to 3 hours
- *Recovery Time:* 2-8 weeks

Pediatric Surgery

- hernia repair
- removal of the appendix (*appendectomy*)
- cancer surgery involving the chest or abdominal cavity
- correct congenital abnormalities of the gastrointestinal tract or other areas of the body
- *Length of Operation:* from 30 minutes for a hernia repair to 5 hours for complex cancer operations
- *Recovery Time:* 1-8 weeks

Plastic and Reconstructive Surgery

- cosmetic surgery (face-lifts, rhinoplasty or "nose job")
- breast reconstruction after cancer surgery (placement of implants or muscle after *mastectomy)*
- trunk and torso surgery *(liposuction,* "tummy tucks," breast augmentation or reduction)
- hand surgery
- skin grafts and repairs for burn victims

- *Length of Operation:* 30 minutes to 4 hours
- *Recovery Time:* 2-8 weeks

Transplant Surgery
- kidney transplants (*renal transplantation*)
- liver transplantation
- corneal (front of the eyeball) transplantation
- heart and lung transplantation
- *Length of Operation:* up to 10 hours
- *Recovery Time:* 6-12 weeks

Urologic Surgery
- removal of a kidney, mainly for cancer (*nephrectomy*)
- examination of the urinary tract with a fiber-optic scope (*cystoscopy*)
- removal of the prostate gland (*prostatectomy*)
- removal of all or part of the bladder (*cystectomy*)
- testicular surgery
- *Length of Operation:* 1 to 4 hours
- *Recovery Time:* 2-8 weeks

Vascular Surgery
- removal of plaque blocking the main arteries in the neck (*carotid endarterectomy*)
- repair of abdominal aortic aneurysm
- leg bypass surgery (use of vein or a tube to bypass blockages in the legs)
- *Length of Operation:* 1-2 hours for a carotid endarterectomy to 8 hours for complex aneurysm or leg bypass surgery
- *Recovery Time:* 2-8 weeks

The types of surgeries are many and varied, ranging from the most minor to a major operation. Even if the type of surgery you've having is listed in this chapter, ask your physician about the length of time it will take to perform your operation and how to plan your recuperation period.

Chapter 7

Your Medical Team

The health care field is comprised of dozens of specialties and subspecialties. In the course of your hospitalization, you will meet a number of health care workers from various fields. The care you receive will be a highly organized effort by a team of health care professionals. They will work to ensure your well-being before, during, and after your surgery. This chapter introduces you to their work.

The Team Approach

Hospitals and health care centers have found that a team approach is the best way to treat patients. Why is this important? A team approach means that more health care professionals will be directly involved in your surgery. They will know firsthand what has happened to you and how well you are responding. Your care will be discussed among a group of people, some of whom may observe key signs and symptoms that others have not seen that could affect your treatment. By using a team approach, a hospital can deliver continuity of care for patients.

Members of the Team

You may be surprised at the number of health care professionals involved directly or indirectly with your case. Many of them you may never see or meet, including supply clerks and medical secretaries. However, during the course of your hospitalization, you will meet many professionals directly involved in your care.

Primary Surgeon

Your *primary surgeon* will perform your operation. If another surgeon is needed, he/she is considered the *second surgeon* or *second scrub*. The term *scrub* comes from the fact that most everyone in the operating room first "scrubs in," or washes, for several minutes to sterilize their skin.

You also may find that your surgeon has one or more surgical assistants in the operating room. These individuals are often surgical residents-in-training who will assist in your procedure as your primary surgeon allows.

As an internist, I work with the rest of the health care team and stay in constant communication until the patient leaves the hospital.

Joseph, 44
Internist

Nurses

Surgical Nurses

There are two types of surgical nurses. A *scrub nurse* scrubs in and assists the surgeon with sterile procedures during your operation. A *circulating nurse* performs other important tasks like retrieving wrapped items from cabinets or relaying information to individuals outside the operating room. Because he/she is not directly involved in the procedure, the circulating nurse also may help ensure that you are comfortable during surgery, especially if you are not under general anesthesia. This nurse may also act as your advocate if you can't communicate certain needs.

Registered Nurse (RN)

Registered nurses (RNs) provide hands-on care. They plan and supervise your nursing care. They also instruct other nursing staff, patients, and their families. RNs have a minimum two-year associate's degree. Many have bachelor's and master's degrees. They also have passed a state board examination. Most nurses in the surgical suite will likely be RNs, as will some if not all of the nurses in the surgeon's and primary care doctor's offices.

Patients expect compassion and competence from us nurses. We do a lot of teaching patients about medications, procedures and tests they may undergo.
Julie, 23
R.N.

Nurse Practitioner (NP)

A *nurse practitioner (NP)* is a registered nurse who has advanced academic and clinical experience. An NP may diagnose and manage many common illnesses. He/she may have a certificate or master's degree in nursing and has completed an internship under the direct supervision of a physician or experienced NP. Practicing under the rules and regulations of their state, NPs may also be nationally certified. In most states they may prescribe medicine.

Licensed Practical Nurse (LPN)

Licensed practical nurses (LPNs) assist nurses with your care in the hospital. They will take your temperature and blood pressure, give you medications, dress wounds, and apply compresses. LPNs have completed one year of nursing school and have passed a state examination to receive their license.

Nursing Aides or Assistants

Nursing aides and *assistants* help with your care under the direct supervision of the nursing staff. They may transport you to and from your room for exams and treatment, serve your meals, take your vital signs, and make your bed. Aides receive training but are not required to be licensed.

Home-Health Nurse or Aide

Your at-home recovery may be aided by visits from a home-health professional. If you will need help with such things as wound dressings, then you will probably see a *home-health nurse.* If you will need assistance with some of your activities of daily living, such as getting dressed, a *home-health aide* will more likely visit you.

> *Patients often expect doctors to have all the answers immediately. But often we don't. In some cases, it can take time to arrive at a diagnosis. Medicine is an art as well as a science.*
>
> *Paul, 70*
> *Retired Physician*

Nurse Anesthetist

A *nurse anesthetist* is a registered nurse trained to assist in the determination, preparation and administration of drugs used for anesthesia. He/she assists the anesthesiologist or gives anesthesia under the doctor's supervision.

Anesthesiologist

An *anesthesiologist* is a medical doctor with special training in delivering anesthetics. He/she will administer your anesthesia and monitor your vital signs while you are under anesthesia. The anesthesiologist is responsible for your medical, not surgical, care in the operating room.

Pathologist

A *pathologist* is a medical doctor who specializes in the examination of cells and tissues to discover disease. For example, if you have had a cyst biopsied, the substance taken from the cyst will be sent to a pathologist. He/she will run various tests to determine if the cyst is benign or malignant.

Pharmacist

A *pharmacist* is responsible for dispensing all your medications. He/she is trained in the science of individual drugs, including their effects and side effects. A pharmacist is not a medical doctor but does have at least five years of specialized college studies.

Primary Care Physician

The initial diagnosis that led you to surgery probably came from your *primary care physician.* A medical doctor, he/she may practice general medicine, family medicine, or internal medicine (*internist*). While you are in the hospital, you will very likely see your primary care physician or an associate. After you leave your surgeon's care, you will return to your primary care physician.

Physician's Assistant

Under the supervision of a physician, a *physician's assistant* helps with a variety of duties—giving physical exams, performing diagnostics, administering therapeutic procedures, and providing education for patients. In addition to a college degree, a physician's assistant receives approximately two years of training in an accredited medical program. Then he/she must pass a national exam to receive certification and the right to practice.

Radiologist

A *radiologist* performs such tests as x-rays, CAT scans, MRIs, and ultrasound. A radiologist will typically examine the test results with the medical team to help diagnose a patient's condition. The radiologist may also recommend additional tests. Note: a radiologist is not involved with radiation therapy to treat cancer; such work is done by a radiation oncologist.

Phlebotomist

A *phlebotomist* is trained to draw blood and prepare samples to be sent to a laboratory for tests ordered by your doctors.

Therapists

Hospitals and other health care centers staff a variety of therapists who may help you recover from surgery.

Physical Therapist

These therapists focus on maximizing one's mobility and independence. They help patients improve walking, balance, strength, leg coordination, and range-of-joint motion. *Physical therapists* also work to reduce any pain you may experience from surgery. Among the tools they use are exercise, massage, ultrasound, heat, cold, and electrical stimulation.

Most patients are worried, particularly after major surgery, about not being able to get around like they used to. My job is to make sure patients are ambulatory enough to take care of themselves at home.

Mike, 33
Physical Therapist

Respiratory Therapist

If you have a problem with your cardiopulmonary system (basically, your heart and lungs) or have been suffering from asthma, pneumonia, bronchitis, or emphysema, you will likely see a *respiratory therapist.* He/she may help you work on your breathing with the aid of different equipment and exercises. This person also works with individuals who must remain on a respirator.

Occupational Therapist

The work of *occupational therapists* involves helping patients regain the ability to perform basic daily activities such as dressing, grooming, and meal preparation. Occupational therapists use a number of techniques to help patients. They often work in environments that resemble bedrooms or kitchens so that patients may relearn how to perform activities of daily living.

Speech Therapist or Speech Pathologist

These professionals evaluate patients' ability to speak and comprehend what is being said to them. If the patients are experiencing a deficit in these areas, the therapists design strategies to help them restore language skills and learn other ways to communicate, if necessary.

Audiologist

Trained to identify and prevent hearing problems, *audiologists* assist with the rehabilitation of patients whose problems involve hearing.

Prosthetist and Orthotist

A *prosthetist* makes and adjusts artificial limbs and teaches you how to use a prosthetic device. An *orthotist* makes braces and splints for limbs and other orthotic devices.

Social Workers

The goal of *social workers* is to ensure that patients have the skills and services they need once they leave the hospital. They also help solve unexpected problems related to a patient's hospitalization, from overcoming depression to logistics, such as needing a ride home.

Dietitian

Also called *nutritionists*, hospital *dietitians* are responsible for meal planning, making sure that all your meals are balanced and nutritious. They also plan special menus for patients who are on restricted diets. Dieticians often counsel patients on healthful cooking and eating habits at home.

> *Many patients have trouble breathing after major surgery and I use my skills to get their lungs back in working order. By the time I am done with patients, they are breathing a lot easier.*
>
> *Stephanie, 29*
> *Respiratory therapist*

Technicians and Technologists

A number of technicians are always busy assisting other health care workers. They may prepare equipment and administer tests or therapies. The operating room, for example, may be set up by the very technician who will also help with your care during surgery. If you have an X-ray taken or are having radiation treatment, you may be helped by a *radiation therapy technologist*. Similarly, you may meet a *cardiovascular technologist* if you are having heart tests, such as an echocardiogram. In the area of nuclear medicine, which uses electromagnetic radiation to image organs for diagnosis, both technicians and technologists play a role in preparing and administering solutions with the radioactive substances.

Chapter 8

Preparing for Surgery

Depending on your diagnosis, you may have days or weeks in which to prepare for surgery. Whichever the case, your doctor will probably order laboratory tests prior to your operation. Often, these tests will be done at the hospital where your operation is scheduled.

Tests may be noninvasive, in that no incisions are made during the testing, or invasive, during which a needle or other instrument will enter your body. Examples of noninvasive tests include X-rays, urine analysis, scans (like ultrasound and magnetic resonance imaging), and an electrocardiogram. Procedures such as catheterization and angiography of the heart and even drawing blood are invasive tests. Fortunately, advanced testing technologies have eliminated the need for exploratory surgery in some instances. Your physician may order tests from among the list that follows.

Medical Tests

Blood Tests

- Normally, two or three small tubes of blood will be taken from you several days before surgery. Blood tests are usually performed to determine (1) whether there are any changes in the normal parts of your blood and (2) whether there is anything abnormal in your blood. The most common blood tests check the following:
- the number of red and white blood cells (a complete blood count, or CBC)
- the distribution of the different types of white blood cells (which fight infection), the size, shape and amount of hemoglobin (the part that carries oxygen) in the red blood cells
- proportions of magnesium, sodium, potassium, and other electrolytes
- how well your blood clots
- how well your liver is working and whether there are any enzymes of the type released when heart or liver tissue is damaged

The surgeon and the anesthesiologist want to make sure all these values are within the normal range before you are given sedation or general anesthesia.

Urine analysis

This test will reveal whether you have a kidney or bladder infection, which may exist if you complain of burning or pain, urinate frequently, or have pain in your side next to your kidney.

Pregnancy test

If you are a woman of childbearing age, you may have a pregnancy test. If a specific protein is found in the blood or urine, then you are pregnant. Medically and legally, it is necessary to document the presence or lack of a pregnancy since many medications given during an operation could harm a developing fetus. If the test is unexpectedly positive, your surgeon will likely cancel your surgery to discuss your options.

X-rays

Produced by low levels of radiation, *X-rays* are photographic images of the inside of your body. The lower the density of the material being photographed, the more transparent it appears on the final picture or film. This is why bones and cartilage show up very clearly in X-rays, and also why X-rays help detect tumors in soft tissue. To get better pictures of softer tissues or structures, the radiologist or radiology technician may have you swallow *contrast media* to help outline internal structures. However, if no particular problems are suspected, you will probably only have a chest X-ray prior to surgery.

My surgeon was nice enough to let me know that all the blood tests before the operation were normal. He also informed me why they were needed and what they all meant.

Steve, 39
Patient

Electrocardiogram (ECG or EKG)

Electrodes are attached to your chest to read the electrical currents created when your heart beats. The electrode wires are attached to an *electrocardiograph*, which traces the impulse onto a special piece of paper; these tracings are the ECG. Based on peaks, valleys, and other irregularities in the tracings, doctors may determine whether your heart rhythm is normal. They may also tell if the heart chambers are enlarged, if your heartbeat is stronger or weaker than what would be considered normal, and more. An ECG may be given to you either lying down or walking on a treadmill.

Ultrasound

A high-frequency sound wave is projected into the body, sending back different signals depending on the density of the tissue it hits. A computer produces a two-dimensional picture from the signals. Because an *ultrasound* is considered very safe, it is often used on pregnant women. This scan is also used to examine organs filled with fluid, such as the gall bladder, and other structures, such as the liver and kidneys. An advanced form of ultrasound, *Doppler ultrasound*, is very effective in showing how fast blood flows through the arteries of the heart.

Computerized Axial Tomography (CAT) Scan

CAT scans, also referred to as CT (*computerized tomography*) scans, rely on X-ray detectors arranged in a semicircle. CAT scans take two-dimensional pictures of "slices" of the body, and a three-dimensional image is built from those slices. These scans help in the study of soft tissue, showing much better resolution than X-rays.

Positron Emission Tomography (PET) Scan

Positrons, which are simply positively charged particles, are injected into the body with a radioactive substance. The positrons release another particle that is detected by a scanner to produce images to evaluate chemical and metabolic activity in the brain and heart. These help to detect tumors and to investigate stroke damage to the brain, Parkinson's disease, epilepsy, and hardening of the arteries.

Magnetic Resonance Imaging (MRI)

Instead of radiation, an MRI uses a strong magnetic field and radio waves to slightly move the atoms in your body. The movement gives off radio signals that the MRI scanner's computer translates into an image. Like PET and CAT scans, an MRI is done in a machine with a circular opening. You lie down on a padded board that moves you into the machine. You may feel claustrophobic. If so, discuss this fully with your surgeon.

Endoscopy

Endoscopy is more involved than other tests, in that you are usually given a sedative beforehand because the fiber-optic scope may produce pain and discomfort. Different scopes have been developed to view different parts the body, and most may be inserted without any incisions. For example, an endoscope may be passed through the mouth down to the stomach, lungs, and even the intestines. (The intestines may also be viewed with a *colonoscope*, which is inserted through the rectum.)

Most patients usually need lab tests before surgery. Many patients never learn the results. My job is to alert the doctors to any abnormal test results so the necessary measures can be taken.

Mary Jo, 39
Nurse

Angiography and Cardiac Catheterization

These two tests involve blood vessels and the heart. For both, an incision is first made, usually in the groin. Then a guide-wire is inserted into an artery and threaded to the appropriate area using

X-ray screening to follow its progress. A thin tube called a *catheter* is then threaded along the wire, which is removed when the catheter is in place.

With *angiography*, a contrast fluid is injected through the catheter, and the fluid outlines the arteries. A video is made of the process, later to be studied for blockages or other problems in the blood vessels.

With *cardiac catheterization*, the catheter passes into the heart itself. This allows doctors to:
- better see the heart
- take blood samples to analyze how well the heart circulates the blood
- decide how well heart valves are working by taking measurements of blood pressure
- inject drugs directly into the area needed to dissolve clots
- try to open blocked arteries with small balloons (*angioplasty*) or by inserting a stent, a small mesh tube.

Electroencephalogram (EEG)

Electrodes are attached to the skull to trace the brain's electrical activity. The patterns of the tracings may reveal a brain tumor or injury, internal bleeding, brain inflammation, or other conditions.

Other tests may involve getting tissue or fluid samples for laboratory analysis. All test results are sent to your surgeon's office. You may want to call to learn the results. This information may help better prepare you for surgery. Also, if blood tests indicate abnormal levels of various substances, your surgeon may want you to take certain drugs or supplements to balance the levels.

Other Preparations

Medications

You and your surgeon should discuss in detail what to do about all the medications you are taking prior to your surgery, including both over-the-counter medications and prescription drugs. In some cases, you may be asked to stop taking certain medications prior to surgery. Other times, you may be told to continue a prescription. There is no single answer when it comes to dealing with your medications prior to surgery. That is why it is crucial to discuss all medications with your surgeon.

Create a Health Journal

Whenever you meet with the surgeon or other health care professionals, you might consider taking a health journal with you. Most of us don't have one. But if you are facing surgery, it is an excellent idea to create one.

Essentially, a health journal catalogs your medical history as far back as you can remember or have records to document. You should write in reverse chronological order; that is, list the most recent events first. Helpful information would include:

- past/present conditions or problems
- your age when dealing with each problem
- doctors consulted, with contact information
- tests conducted and the results
- treatments
- description of recovery and recuperation
- medications/drug treatment for each problem
- list of allergies, if any
- outcome of each illness or hospitalization

This journal should be as complete as possible. Include your thoughts and feelings, because they will impact your upcoming surgery. If you've had good experiences, you will probably be less anxious than if you've never had surgery or, worse yet, if you've had a bad surgical experience.

Advance Directive

In an *advance directive*, a legally binding document, you specify how you wish to be cared for if you are incapacitated and can't make your own decisions. While most of us don't like thinking about this possibility, it is wise to make decisions while you rationally can. It may save you and your family a great deal of worry, pain, and expense if ever your recovery is questionable. There are essentially two types of advance directives.

Before patients leave my office, I tell them what tests are coming prior to their surgery. As long as they know what is needed, they feel much less anxious about the whole experience.
Tony, 42, M.D.
Surgeon

A *living will* states exactly what kind of health care you do or don't want under specific circumstances. For example, you may want all measures taken to keep you alive, or you may decide you want no measures taken at all. Keep a copy of your living will handy.

In addition, you will find an Internet service (www.uslivingwillregistry.com) through which you may register your living will. This service ensures that your living will is available at all times.

A *durable health care power of attorney* (also called a *health care proxy*) lets you designate an individual to make decisions about your health care if you cannot. You should discuss this option thoroughly with whomever you name and make sure the person is aware of your health-care preferences. Still, you should consider drafting a living will, because it will be of great help to the person holding your health-care proxy. Check the laws of your state governing both advance directives.

Organ Donation

Another area that you may have already considered is *organ donation*. You may already have a donor card. If not, you may get one from the U.S. Health Resources and Services Administration or the U.S. Department of Health and Human Services from the Internet site http://www.organdonor.gov.

Both the person holding your durable health care power of attorney and the hospital administration should be aware of your wishes regarding organ donation.

Autologous Blood Donation

Many people heading into major surgery have concerns about needing blood transfusions. You may discuss this possibility with your surgeon. If you are concerned about the blood supply at the hospital, you may have time to donate your own blood to be held for your surgery. This is called *autologous blood donation.*

To make this kind of donation, you schedule a time at the hospital's blood bank to donate blood. You should discuss with your surgeon the best time to make this donation if there are concerns about a reduced blood supply circulating in your system.

It is not necessary that you donate blood for yourself. The techniques used to screen blood today are highly sophisticated, making transfusion a safer prospect than ever before.

The Admissions Process

Most hospitals today allow you to visit the admissions office to get paperwork started before you are actually admitted. You will be asked to fill out many forms.

When you go to the admissions office, always take proof of your health insurance with you. This is very important. If you have no proof of insurance, you will be expected to pay for your entire surgery and hospital stay. In fact, most insurance companies require you to get approval for your surgery before you ever have an operation. This process is usually done by staff in your surgeon's office, although HMOs and other such plans have their own procedures. If your surgeon's staff has not gotten approval for your surgery, you need to call them to find out why.

An admissions staff member will provide the forms for you to fill out. Some hospitals keep these together in a packet.

General Information Form

This form requests essential patient information such as name, address, next of kin, insurance company, and physician. The completed form stays on your medical chart during your entire hospital experience.

Health Questionnaire

With this form, you tell the hospital about your medical history (including allergies and smoking history), medications, previous surgeries, previous complications, and the like. It also contains a list of diseases and asks you to check off the ones you've had.

Surgical Consent Form

All patients have to sign this form before their operation. Because it is a legal document that goes in your medical file, you should read it thoroughly and make sure you understand it. It is usually a one-page document naming your condition, the procedure to be done (described both in plain English and medical terms), and who will perform it. The form also states that you completely understand the risks and benefits of the operation to be carried out. If these risks and benefits have not been fully explained to you, do not sign the form. Normally a nurse witness, sometimes two, will verify your acknowledgment of understanding and cosign the form.

Good Self-Care

A healthy lifestyle will help you get through surgery with less pain and recover more quickly. When you're tired and stressed, eating on the run, and not sleeping enough, your body may get run down. You can't spring back as well from setbacks, be they physical or emotional.

Prior to my leaving my surgeon's office, a nurse gave me a list of things to do the day before my operation. This was extremely helpful. Taking notes also helped me.

Dottie, 45
Patient

Remember, if your lifestyle is less than healthy, trying to make changes just before surgery won't guarantee a super-fast recovery. Still, making an effort should help. Be as healthy as you can be.

Diet

Eat balanced, nutritious meals. This means less fat and sugar, more fiber and carbohydrates. Choose whole-grain breads,

A Patient's Bill of Rights

This document, adopted by the American Hospital Association in 1973, outlines your rights to receive considerate care, information, privacy, and more, as well as your right to make decisions about your care and to refuse treatment. It will help you understand your rights while in the hospital and that you have a responsibility to be involved in your well-being. The bill comprises the following twelve points:

1. The patient has the right to considerate and respectful care.

2. The patient has the right to obtain from caregivers relevant, current, and understandable information concerning diagnosis, treatment, and prognosis. This includes information related to specific procedures and/or treatments, risks involved, length of recuperation, and medically reasonable alternatives and their risks and benefits. Patients have the right to know the identity of everyone involved in their care, as well as when those involved are students or trainees. The patient also has the right to know the financial implications of treatment choices, insofar as they are known.

3. The patient has the right to make decisions about the plan of care prior to and during treatment and to refuse a recommended treatment or plan of care to the extent permitted by law and hospital policy. If a patient refuses recommended treatment, the patient is still entitled to other care and services within that hospital or to be transferred to another hospital.

4. The patient has the right to have an advance directive and to expect that the hospital will honor that directive to the extent permitted by law and hospital policy. The patient has the right to know whether and how a hospital's policies limit its ability to fully implement a legally valid advance directive.

5. The patient has the right to every consideration of privacy. Case discussion, consultation, examination, and treatment should be conducted so as to protect each patient's privacy.

6. The patient has the right to expect that all communications and records pertaining to his/her care will be treated as confidential by the hospital, except when law requires or permits reporting, such as suspected abuse and public health hazards. The hospital should emphasize the information's confidentiality when released to other parties entitled to review the patient's records.

7. The patient has the right to review records pertaining to his/her medical care and to have the information explained or interpreted as necessary, except when restricted by law.

8. The patient has the right to expect that, within its capacity and policies, a hospital will reasonably respond to a patient's request for appropriate and medically indicated care and services, which may include being transferred to another facility. The hospital must provide evaluation, service, and/or referral as indicated by a case's urgency. The patient must also have complete information concerning the need for risks, benefits, and alternatives to a transfer.

9. The patient has the right to ask and be informed of the existence of business relationships among the hospital, educational institutions, other health care providers, or payers that may influence the patient's treatment and care.

10. The patient has the right to consent to or decline to participate in research studies or human experimentation affecting care and treatment or requiring direct patient involvement, and to have those studies fully explained prior to consent. A patient who declines to participate is entitled to the most effective care that the hospital can otherwise provide.

11. The patient has the right to expect reasonable continuity of care when appropriate and to be informed by caregivers of available and realistic patient care options when hospital care is no longer appropriate.

12. The patient has the right to be informed of hospital policies and practices that relate to patient care, treatment, and responsibilities, as well as the right to be informed of available resources for resolving disputes and grievances, such as patient representatives, and any charges related to these services.

cereals, and pastas; vegetables; fruits; low-fat or skim dairy products; soy products; and lots of water. Meat selections should include fish and poultry, and if you eat red meat, make it lean. A daily glass or two of wine has been found to help your heart, so don't feel you can't have any. However, too much wine or other alcohol will only hurt, not help.

Vitamins and supplements

A healthy diet should provide most of the vitamins and minerals your body requires each day. Still, it may be a good idea to take a complete multivitamin and possibly other supplements, with the approval of your physician.

Exercise

If you have not been on a regular exercise program, you should never suddenly begin one without your doctor's approval. Still even gentle exercise will give your body a boost. Ask your doctor about an exercise program. How many minutes each day should you exercise? What type of activity should you do? Remember that exercise does not have to be exhausting. For example, thirty minutes of walking per day may be divided into two segments, fifteen minutes each.

Emotional / Spiritual

The sooner your surgery, the more anxious you may become. This is normal. Don't criticize yourself for feeling worried. You don't need the additional stress. Continual stress only works against you. Studies have shown the negative effects of stress on the body. For example, one study has found that stress may dangerously raise levels of a substance in the body called *homocysteine*, which damages artery walls and causes plaque to build up in those arteries.

Engage in whatever activity will help you relax. If you have a relaxation tape, use it as often as you need. Visualization is also helpful. It involves mental imagery—seeing events unfold in a positive way in your mind's eye. At least one study has shown that visualization boosts immunity. Athletes use visualization to help them attain their goals. You may use it to gain the best possible results from surgery and to promote faster, less painful recovery. The imagery you select should be bright and positive. Do not focus on the actual surgical process. Instead, think about the end result of the surgery and picture your return to health. Imagine yourself healthy and happy in pleasant surroundings.

Chapter 9

The Night Before Surgery

On the night before surgery, you will probably be somewhat anxious. This is natural. Don't be self-critical over the fact that you're worried or frightened. Instead, concentrate on what you need to do to be ready in the morning. The more organized you are, the less stress you'll likely feel. This is a good time to review your list of things to do prior to leaving for the hospital. Confirm the time you'll leave for the hospital with your spouse, family member, friend, or whomever will be taking you.

Packing for the Hospital

The length of your stay in the hospital should help you decide what you need to take. The longer your stay, the more you may wish to take. If you are staying only one night, you'll need pajamas or a nightgown (the looser the better), a robe, slippers, underwear, and clothes to wear when you leave the hospital. These clothes, like those you wear to the hospital (they may be the same outfit), should be easy to put on and take off. Sweatshirts, sweatpants, drawstring pants or shorts, T-shirts, and shifts are ideal. After surgery, your movement may be restricted. You may not be able to handle buttons, zippers, and belts. You also may find that fitted clothes are uncomfortable, depending on where your incision is.

Other personal items you may wish to pack:

- toothbrush
- mouthwash
- hairbrush
- creams
- soap
- toothpaste
- dental floss
- razor
- shampoo

If you are taking medications, you should not take your own supply. Instead, your surgeon will order the medications you will receive while in the hospital. Be sure your surgeon is aware of every prescription you currently take. He/she may stop one or more of your daily medications during your recovery, especially if those drugs could interfere with other medications you need to help you heal.

You may wish to take books or magazines, a sheet with phone numbers and addresses if you want to make calls, stationery for writing letters, puzzles, or handcrafts. You may also take a portable radio or cassette/CD player, but remember your headphones in case your roommate's taste in music or audiobooks doesn't match yours. You may also take a laptop computer. However, it is an unfortunate fact of hospital life that items disappear. If you do take something valuable like a computer, you may want to ask a family member to take it home at night. Also, most hospitals frown on patients plugging electrical cords into the walls, so make sure everything you take is battery operated.

Some items you should definitely leave at home. Leave behind your wedding ring, watches, and other jewelry. These could be lost or stolen. Also, leave behind your artificial nails or nail polish. This is important. Nurses often evaluate your blood circulation simply by checking the color of your fingernail beds. Remove your polish or artificial nails before entering the hospital. You want to give your surgical team every advantage in making sure you are doing fine throughout your hospital visit.

Fasting and Diet

No matter what your surgery, you probably will be told not to eat or drink anything after midnight the night before the scheduled operation. Because your stomach takes anywhere from six to eight hours to empty itself of food, a midnight cutoff means your stomach should be cleared out by the time you undergo surgery. You may consider eating a lighter dinner the night before your surgery and stop eating earlier than midnight.

I explain to patients what special instructions need to be followed prior to their operation. I make sure everything is written down and understood before they leave the doctor's office.

Carol, 54
Nurse

Having an empty stomach is especially important if you are having general anesthesia because you lose control of several reflex functions. This includes the *gag reflex* that keeps food and stomach acid from rising up in your throat and possibly into your lungs. This can create serious problems, including a life-threatening illness called *asphyxiation pneumonia*. A breathing tube may block this reflux material, but this hazard may be avoided simply by following your surgeon's instructions to fast after a certain hour.

In addition to fasting, you may be asked to have only a liquid diet the entire day before surgery. This is most likely if your surgery involves any organ of the digestive tract or the abdomen. A liquid diet helps speed up digestion and move waste products through the intestines faster. Don't think that a liquid diet means having nothing at all. You need fluids to help keep your digestive tract moving and to prevent dehydration.

If your surgeon decides you need to completely empty your digestive tract, he/she will prescribe a liquid laxative that should be taken according to instructions provided by a pharmacist. These laxatives usually don't taste very good, but they are very effective. Once they start working, it's a good idea to stay close to the bathroom.

Medications

If you are currently on medication, your surgeon or a member of his/her staff will tell you which one(s) to take up to the time of surgery. Always get these directions in writing. Make sure you are absolutely clear about what you should be doing. Depending on your surgery or your condition, your surgeon may order new medications for you to take for a certain amount of time.

When your anesthesiologist decides how much anesthesia to use for your surgery, he/she considers not only your weight and allergies but also the medications you are currently taking. This is another important reason to follow your physician's instructions carefully.

Many over-the-counter medicines also may create problems during your surgery. You will be told not to take them. For example, aspirin and other so-called anti-inflammatory medications tend to thin your blood and should be stopped a week to ten days before your operation. If not, your tendency to bleed will increase and could complicate your surgery. If you are taking any other blood-thinning medications, such as warfarin, stop taking them prior to surgery. If you have been taking any blood-thinning medications, your surgeon probably will order a blood test right before surgery to determine whether your blood is clotting normally.

If you are a diabetic, it is likely that you will be told not to take insulin the morning of surgery. With no food or drink in your stomach because you've been fasting, a shot of insulin could cause the glucose level in your blood to drop dangerously low. Again, ask your surgeon if you have any doubts about your medications.

Hygiene

Unless otherwise instructed, you should be able to shower or bathe normally the night before surgery. Consider how soothing a warm bath would be. If you're at home the night before, you might consider putting on relaxing music, adding some bubbles or oils, and letting yourself relax for some time.

The biggest fear most patients have right before they enter the operating room is the fear of the unknown—not knowing what to expect. Commonly, as patients are wheeled into the operating room they tell me, 'please, take good care of me.'

Brian, 31
Operating Room R.N.

Regular shaving—facial hair for men and leg hair for women—is allowed. However, do not shave near the area where your surgeon will be operating. You will need to be shaved if your surgery involves an area of your body that is covered in hair, such as your head, your groin, even your chest or abdomen. Although you may feel more comfortable shaving at home, leave it to the health care professionals. You could cut or nick yourself. An open wound could become infected. Your surgical team knows exactly what area needs to be shaved and can do so more precisely to better prepare you for surgery.

Sexual Relations

You may be embarrassed to ask whether it's okay to have sex the night before your operation. Generally speaking, it's okay. After your operation, it may be some time before you can resume sexual intimacy. For instance, just after a hernia operation, sexual intercourse may be too painful. Your surgeon may recommend a few weeks of abstinence.

If you have concerns about sexual activity, discuss them openly with your surgeon. A medical professional, your surgeon has been asked these questions many times.

Getting to Sleep

Get a good night's sleep before your operation. It's one of the best things you can do. This is a good time to use any techniques that in the past have helped you to fall asleep. A warm glass of milk, soothing music, relaxation techniques, or exercise during the day may help you drift off to sleep.

If you anticipate being quite anxious the night before surgery, you may want to talk to your surgeon about taking a mild sedative. However, avoid over-the-counter sleeping pills without first consulting your surgeon. Again, one pill may not seem like much, but it could interact with other medications that have been ordered for your surgery.

Chapter 10

Checking in at the Hospital

The time for your surgery is drawing near. Depending on your type of surgery, you will either check into the hospital the day before or the day of your operation. If you have already gone through a preadmissions process, you may have little to do when you visit the admissions office, other than to sign last-minute paperwork. It is a good idea to carry with you all the papers you have already completed. During check-in, be sure to ask for copies of anything else you need to sign.

Checking In

If this is your first time visiting the admissions office for surgery, you will have many forms to fill out. If you can't get to the hospital before check-in day, you should call to learn how long the admissions process will take. Always allow yourself enough time to finish everything.

During check-in, you will get an identification bracelet that lists your name, your hospital identification number, possibly your admitting physician's name, and any known drug allergies. Don't take this off before you leave the hospital. Hospital staff rely on this bracelet to correctly identify patients.

Once you are finished in the admissions office, if your operation is scheduled for today, you will be taken (possibly in a wheelchair) to a room where preparations for your operation will get underway. Any family members accompanying you probably will be allowed to stay with you at this point.

If you are checking in a day or more before your surgery so that you can undergo preoperative testing as an inpatient, you will likely be taken to a regular room in the hospital. This may or may not be the room you eventually return to after your operation. By now you should have a thorough idea of the tests you will undergo and your schedule during the day. If you don't, ask the nurse overseeing your care.

Your Hospital Chart

Your hospital chart is a vital record that documents your medical history, including results from tests you took prior to coming to the hospital. Medical personnel from nearly every department will use your chart as a guide to your progress. It details measurements, test results, and observations that will be recorded during your hospitalization. It also will contain copies of documents you have signed, including a surgical consent form.

This is *your* chart. You have the right to read it. Still, few patients ask to see their charts. Don't be surprised if the hospital staff checks your request with your doctor before giving it to you. Ask your physician to note in your chart that you may read it if you wish.

Heading to the Operating Room

Before entering the operating room, you will be asked to change into a hospital gown. You will also be asked to remove any jewelry, dentures, or contact lenses. Depending on the amount of time that has passed since you first talked with a nurse, you may have your blood pressure, heart rate, and temperature taken again at least once, if not several times. Another nurse or phlebotomist may draw blood if your surgeon or anesthesiologist has ordered it. While this is not typical, your test results may prompt your doctors to seek up-to-date information.

Unless your hospital has a no-visitor policy, your family should still be able to remain with you at this point. The presence of loved ones should bring comfort if you find yourself growing anxious.

Delays in getting you into the operating room are always possible. Sometimes delays cannot be avoided. They usually have little to do with your operation. If your surgeon is late, it is likely for one of two reasons. He/she may be performing an emergency procedure on another patient, or the operation prior to yours is taking longer than was expected.

When patients arrive on the morning of their surgery, they can become overwhelmed with admissions paper work. I try to take them through each step slowly, making sure all questions are answered and understood.

Edith, 44
Nurse

Once most of these preparations are complete, you may have a chance to talk to a member of the anesthesiology team to learn more about the anesthesia that will be used during your operation.

Chapter 11

Anesthesia

When it comes time to deliver anesthesia, your care will pass into the hands of an anesthesiologist. This physician will have decided which anesthesia to give you, having reviewed your medical history, including previous operations, allergies, current medications, and any previous problems with anesthesia. A variety of techniques are used to deliver anesthesia. How you receive anesthesia may depend, in part, on the kind of surgery you're having. Some methods are preferred for certain operations.

Types of Anesthesia

General Anesthesia

In many cases, the medical team will administer *general anesthesia* which numbs your entire body for the entire time of the surgery. You will be unconscious under a general anesthetic. Accordingly, activity in your brain will slow, as will your heart and breathing. Most major and some minor surgeries are performed under a general anesthetic, especially if the head, neck, chest, or upper abdomen is involved.

Regional Anesthesia

With *regional anesthesia,* an entire region of the body is numbed—an arm, a leg, or the entire body below the waist. Regional anesthesia is often considered safer than general anesthesia for patients with special conditions, including pregnancy and advanced heart disease. It is also an alternative for patients who wish not to be asleep during surgery.

Regional blocks that numb the entire lower half of your body and involve the spinal column are called *epidurals* and *spinals.* For both, the anesthesiologist numbs a spot on your back and inserts a very thin needle. If you are having an epidural, the needle stops just outside the membrane surrounding the spinal column. For a spinal, the needle stops just inside that same membrane. Then the drugs are released into your body. This blocks pain in both instances, but with a spinal, you also lose feeling in your legs. With an epidural, a thin tube is inserted before the needle is removed so that more drugs may be given if needed during the operation.

My anesthesiologist explained everything several days before my surgery. After waking up from the operation, the sick feeling I had and all those tubes attached were not a surprise. I knew what to expect.

Verba, 36
Patient

A spinal anesthetic is a good choice for many operations done below the waist, such as procedures involving hernias, bones, joints, and even major blood vessels. For the surgeon, it ensures that these limbs will not move during the operation. Epidurals are effective if the surgery may last a while and additional anesthesia needs to be given. They also are excellent for women in labor.

Intravenous Sedation with Local Injection

You may have heard of *twilight sedation* or *twilight sleep.* This is another form of anesthesia in which less powerful sedatives are given through an intravenous line. You go to sleep, still breathing on your own, and then a local anesthetic is injected. You won't feel the shot or the operation. This method is used for many outpatient procedures, such as the removal of a breast lump. It produces fewer side effects than does general anesthesia.

I met my anesthesiologist the day of my surgery. It all happened so fast. I wish I would have met him several days before being wheeled into the operating room.

Alison, 35
Patient

Local Anesthesia

Anesthesia that is limited to one part of the body is called *local anesthesia.* It is usually given by injection. Initially, the shot may sting slightly, but the drug quickly numbs the area. Local anesthetic agents (most of which end in the suffix *-caine*) block the nerves from telling the brain that there is pain at the surgery site. Local anesthesia acts for only a short time and is used for suturing cuts, removing warts and moles, and skin biopsies.

Under local anesthesia, you will be awake and aware during your surgery. You may feel pressure at the operation site, which is normal. However, if you should start to feel pain during a procedure, immediately ask the anesthesiologist to give you more anesthesia. The anesthetic should eliminate the pain. Don't think that you have to stoically endure a painful surgery. It is not normal and may be avoided.

Questions to Ask Your Anesthesiology Team

You may have visited with the anesthesiologist or nurse anesthetist prior to your surgery. On the other hand, you may not have the chance to meet the anesthesiologist until just before your operation. In either case, you will probably have questions you'd like answered.

- What kind of anesthesia will you be using? How does it work?
- How will you give it to me? Through a breathing mask or by intravenous line?
- Will I be completely unconscious? Will I remember anything?
- What if I feel pain? What if I feel cutting or tugging? How can I tell you these things?
- Will tubes be inserted in my body? If so, where? Their purpose?
- How will I feel when I wake up?
- Will I be able to breathe on my own, or will I be on a respirator after surgery?
- Are complications possible with the drugs you will be using? If so, what are they? How might you deal with them?

Typically, patients do not choose their anesthesiologist; however, it is possible to do so. If you do wish to have a specific anesthesiologist attending you, it's best to make your wishes known in advance. Otherwise, your surgeon will arrange for the services of one with who he/she is familiar.

Chapter 12

The Operating Room

If you are being taken to an operating suite from a regular hospital room, you will first be taken to the "pre-op" area on a *gurney*, a wheeled bed. You'll likely stay on the gurney until you reach the surgical suite, where you will be moved to an operating table. If family members have been allowed in the pre-op area, they will be able to stay as long as hospital policy permits. Then they will be directed to a waiting area and told when they will receive updates on your surgery.

The nurses in pre-op will make a final check of your hospital chart, reviewing laboratory results, X-rays, and other tests completed earlier. During your time in pre-op, an intravenous line (IV) will likely be started. A small, hollow needle with a hole in its tip will be inserted into a vein, probably in your arm or the top of your hand. The needle is attached to a thin, plastic tube through which medications, fluids, and even anesthetics may flow. You'll probably feel a slight sting when the needle is first inserted, but the discomfort usually disappears quickly.

Because most patients are nervous prior to surgery, surgeons and anesthesiologists often direct nurses to give sedatives or antianxiety medications through the IV line. Even if you are not nervous, a sedative may simply relax you, which will help your surgeon and the rest of the team do their jobs more smoothly. Depending on the type of surgery you are having, nurses may also insert other IV lines that will help your surgical team get fluids into your system as needed. A catheter may also be inserted into your urethra so that your bladder may drain.

You also may receive an antacid, usually taken orally, to reduce the risk of stomach acid coming up during surgery and entering your lungs. Any acid reflux could damage your lungs, complicating your surgery and recovery.

If your surgeon believes there is any risk of infection, he/she will also ensure that you receive an antibiotic. This may be given in the operating room after anesthesia has been administered rather than in pre-op. Antibiotics are commonly used during intestinal surgery because the intestines contain large amounts of bacteria.

When I am operating, I focus on the operation at hand and what I need to do to make this patient well.

Mark, 45, M.D.
Surgeon

The Operating Suite

Once you have received all presurgery medications and the nurses have received the go-ahead from the anesthesiologist, you will be taken on the gurney into the operating room, or operating suite, as some hospitals prefer to call them. If you have seen surgery being conducted on a television show or in a movie, then you will have some idea as to what the room looks like. Most operating rooms are very bright in appearance, largely because they are very well lighted. The entire suite is also kept sterile through rigorous cleaning after each operation.

Once inside, you will be helped from the gurney onto a narrow operating table in the center of the room. The stainless-steel table is usually cold, so a blanket is in order. Don't hesitate to ask for a blanket if no one covers you. If you need to be in a different position than lying flat on your back—for example, if your surgeon will be working on your side or back—you may be helped into the proper position now, or you may be moved into that position after you fall asleep. Depending on the type of surgery, nurses may place a wide strap slightly above your waist to help secure you on the table.

In the V.A. hospital where I work, men are quite often embarrassed about being exposed during their surgery, especially if they are awake. I reassure them that the O.R. is very private and that no one but medical professionals will be in the room.

Becky, 46
Surgical R.N.

Next to the operating table, another table covered by a cloth holds sterilized surgical instruments that the scrub nurse hands to the surgeon during the procedure. Various supplies like bandages, suture equipment, and instruments are usually stored in cabinets along the wall.

You may notice television monitors in the room. These monitors are used during laparascopic surgeries. In some cases, surgeons may videotape their surgeries for teaching purposes.

Close by the operating table, machines are set up to monitor vital functions while you are under anesthesia. Wires from a heart monitor will be attached to your chest, while a blood-pressure cuff will be placed on your upper arm. A *pulse oximeter*, a device that measures the amount of oxygen in your blood, fits on one finger.

A wire from another machine, a *peripheral nerve stimulator*, may be placed lower on your chest to check whether the muscle relaxants you will be given are working. If your surgeon knows that he/she will use *cautery*, which usually involves using an electric current or heat to stop bleeding, then a grounding pad for the machine will be placed on your side near your waist.

A mask, through which oxygen flows, will be fitted over your nose and mouth. A respirator will be nearby in case you need a machine to breathe for you—deliver oxygen to and remove carbon dioxide from your lungs—during the operation. A rack with bags of liquids also will be at the ready to hook into your IV line that was inserted in pre-op. These bags may contain anesthetics and saline solution; the saline in the veins helps maintain blood pressure and assists in the delivery of medications.

Going to Sleep

The anesthesiologist is now ready to give the anesthesia. As the anesthesia enters your body, you will simply fall asleep within seconds.

If you are having twilight sedation, you will be breathing on your own. But if you are under general anesthesia, you will have a breathing tube from a respirator placed down your throat to breathe for you during the operation. The anesthesiologist programs the machine to give the proper amount of oxygen based on your height and weight. Anesthetic gases also may be delivered through the breathing tube as needed during your surgery. The breathing tube has advantages over a mask. It has a small balloon on the end that may be inflated to keep food particles and fluids from your stomach from entering your lungs. It also keeps higher levels of oxygen in your blood than you might otherwise get breathing on your own since your breathing is slowed by the anesthesia.

Many patients also have a catheter placed in their bladder to measure urine output during surgery, especially if the operation is long. A plastic tube may also be placed down a patient's nose, into the stomach, once he/she is asleep. This keeps the stomach empty during major abdominal operations.

Finally, your skin in the surgical area will be shaved and thoroughly cleaned. At the same time, your surgeon will spend at least five minutes scrubbing his/her arms and hands with antibacterial soap. It's time for the operation to begin.

Chapter 13

Surgery Begins

Just moments before the operation begins, your body will be covered with sterile surgical drapes, exposing only the surgery site. These drapes will help keep the transfer of bacteria at the surgical site to a minimum. The drapes will also allow the surgical team to concentrate their full attention on the surgical area.

Making the Incision

Now the surgeon is ready to make the first incision with a *scalpel*. The length of the incision depends on the surgery being performed. If you are having open-heart surgery, for example, a long incision is made down the middle of your chest, giving surgeons access to your heart. For a herniated disk in the lower back, a small incision, only a couple of inches long, may be enough. Scalpels come in different shapes and sizes and are selected according to the body part. All scalpels have one thing in common: they are sharp and will make clean, efficient cuts through skin, muscle, and tissue.

Once the first incision is made, the surgeon continues through layers of skin and muscle as needed to reach the area in which the problem lies. How the rest of your operation is carried out is, of course, dependent on the kind of surgery you're having.

If you have torn ligaments or muscles, they will be sewn back into place. If you're undergoing a joint replacement, cartilage will be cleaned out of the damaged joint, and the joint will be replaced with an artificial one. In heart surgery, the surgeon may have to cut through the sac surrounding the heart as well as the muscle wall itself to reveal internal problems, such as a diseased heart valve that needs to be replaced. If the coronary arteries that sit atop the heart are blocked, other veins may be taken from your leg and sewn onto the obstructed arteries to bypass the blockage, giving your blood a clear channel through which to flow. For cancer patients, surgery usually means removing a tumor. This is always a delicate operation because the goal is to remove the organ invaded by the tumor and leave no cancerous cells behind. Some tumors may be relatively easy to remove. Others may prove more troublesome.

> *The most important part of my job is making the correct diagnosis, pinpointing exactly what is wrong. Once I know this, then I feel confident an operation, if necessary, will make a big difference in the patient's well being.*
> *Steve, 39, M.D.*
> *Surgeon*

Will I Lose Much Blood?

The amount of bleeding depends on how much cutting is done and whether the cut vessels are tiny capillaries or larger veins and arteries. Most bleeding is controlled by cautery. Typically, an electric current coagulates the blood so it stops flowing. If the device applies heat instead of electricity, then it is actually burning blood-vessel tissue to scar the vein shut.

If the bleeding stems from a larger blood vessel, it is clamped shut, cut, and tied off with suture material. If blood flows into a body cavity where your surgeon is working, it will be suctioned out. This suctioning is especially important if the bleeding arises from an unknown source. Removing it will permit the surgeon to see what is bleeding.

Sutures

Once your procedure is completed, your incision, including underlying tissue and muscle, will be sutured shut. There are two categories of sutures: 1) those that dissolve over time and consequently do not have to be removed, and 2) those that must be removed by a surgeon. Suture material comes in all thicknesses and colors. The type chosen by your surgeon depends on the area to be sewn shut. For example, a thicker suture may be used for attaching torn muscles to a shoulder, while a finer suture, one that will cause less scarring, may be used to close a facial incision. For abdominal and chest surgery, staples rather than sutures are often used because they may be inserted quickly.

What I really like about my work is being part of a team, with the ultimate goal of helping make a difference in peoples' lives.

Brian, 30
Operating Room R.N.

In addition to suturing the surgical site, the surgeon may insert one or more tubes in your incision to help drain any excess fluids. Ridding the body of accumulated fluids will help prevent infection.

How Long Will I Be in Surgery?

Your surgeon cannot always answer this question. Often, only an estimate may be given. Assuming you experience no problems during surgery, your surgeon should be able to finish your operation in the amount of time originally estimated. While the operation is underway, the surgeon will probably send out reports to your waiting family and friends. If there are delays or unexpected problems, hopefully your loved ones will be informed as soon as possible.

It is best for the patient if surgery proceeds as quickly as possible. The longer an operation, the greater the risk of complications. For example, prolonged anesthesia could result in one having trouble breathing after the surgery. Or, a long operation could decrease one's body temperature, straining the heart and kidneys.

Today, the speed at which a surgeon performs a specific operation is sometimes taken as one measure of expertise. Operating rooms often track the operating times of surgeons to observe trends and make comparisons. Yet speed does not always mean quality, so your surgeon constantly balances these two elements.

Chapter 14

Possible Complications

Your surgical team is a group of highly trained professionals working with sophisticated technology. But no matter how experienced your surgeon or how well-prepared your surgical team, complications during or after surgery may occur. Sometimes unexpected events lead to complications.

General Complications

Infection

No matter how sterile the operating room, there is always a chance of infection. Some surgeries place patients at a much higher risk of infection. For instance, wound infections and abdominal infections are more common during colon surgery, particularly if colon contents are inadvertently leaked, releasing bacteria. Also, if your surgery is a long one or you lose a lot of blood, you are more likely to suffer a wound infection.

Blood Loss

Some surgeries, especially those involving the heart or major blood vessels, may result in greater blood loss. In other instances, if a blood vessel or organ has been unknowingly cut during surgery, you may experience blood loss. Your surgeon and anesthesiologist will be aware of the problem if excess blood is unexpectedly pooling in a body cavity, or if your blood pressure drops abruptly.

Sometimes bleeding may start after your surgery has ended. Perhaps sutures have come undone or a small nick suddenly enlarges, causing you to bleed internally. You may be taken back to the operating room immediately to have the problem corrected.

Drop in Blood Pressure

Some decrease in blood pressure is expected during surgery, for your heart is pumping more slowly. However, a sudden or continuous drop in blood pressure due to excess blood loss could result in erratic heartbeats or possibly heart attack. Blood pressure is often stabilized by introducing a mineral-rich saline solution into the intravenous line. Other times, a blood transfusion may be necessary to bring blood pressure back up.

Arrhythmia and Other Heart Irregularities

If the heart does not beat normally, one experiences *arrhythmia*. If the heart irregularly speeds up, it is called *atrial fibrillation,* or *flutter.* If the heart regularly slows down, it is called *sinus bradycardia.* If the rhythm is regular but the heartbeat does not come from the proper chambers, it is referred to as *supraventricular tachycardia.* Any of these may occur in the operating room due to stress on your body from the operation and/or the anesthetic. These problems also may result from underlying heart disease or medications that affect you much as caffeine would. If the problem is severe, your surgeon may use a *defibrillator* to administer an electric shock to your heart.

Heart attack

If the stress to your heart is too severe or if the arrhythmias cannot be controlled, you could suffer a heart attack, also known as *myocardial infarction (MI)*. In this event, drugs may be given immediately, some even directly to the heart muscle, to reduce potential damage.

Aspiration

This occurs when you vomit, or *aspirate*, and the vomit is forced up into the lungs. At best this action may prove mildly irritating after you wake up. At worst, it may cause severe infections, a chronic cough, obstruction within the lungs, or pneumonia, all of which may set back your recovery.

Incomplete suturing

If for any reason stitching comes loose, you could experience internal bleeding or a hernia. Should your surgeon determine you are having a suture problem, you may be taken back to the operating room to have the stitches replaced.

Most patients and families experience similar anxieties prior to an operation. This is a very normal thing. Communication between me and the patients before and after an operation is vital toward making the entire experience a positive one.
Paul, 39, M.D.
Surgeon

Human error

Unfortunately, a number of things may go wrong as a result of human mistakes. For example, during surgery a scalpel may accidentally cut tissue that should not have been touched. If your breathing tube was inserted improperly, you may suffer temporary damage to your vocal cords. On the extreme end of error, surgeons have been known to leave sponges or instruments inside patients, requiring additional surgery to remove them. No member of the surgical team intends to inflict such problems, but accidents do happen. This is why it is important to find out everything you can about your surgeon, especially how many times he/she has performed the type of operation you need. The more skilled and experienced the surgeon, the less likely you'll have problems.

Surgeries/Examples of Complications

Every type of surgery carries specific risks due to the nature of the operation. The list of sample complications below is not intended to be alarming, but is intended to give you a better understanding of how a complication can occur. Ask your surgeon for more comprehensive information about the possibilities of complications with your operation.

Thyroidectomy

Behind the thyroid gland, nerves run to the muscles that work the vocal cords. If these are damaged, your voice could be either minimally or seriously altered.

Hysterectomy

The tubes, or *ureters,* that carry urine from the kidneys to the bladder are near the uterus. Should your surgeon injure or somehow cut these structures, urine could leak out, possibly causing an infection. If the ureters are tied off by mistake, urine could back up into the kidneys, causing damage.

Angioplasty

The medical terminology for this procedure is *Percutaneous Transluminal Coronary Angioplasty (PTCA)*. During this operation, a tiny balloon on the end of a tube called a catheter is threaded through the arteries to a place where a blood vessel is blocked. The balloon is gently inflated to unclog the artery. However, if the balloon is overinflated, the arterial wall could be weakened, damaged, or even split. If the split is small, a metal tube called a stent might be threaded up the catheter to seal the tear. However, if the break is large, you would be taken immediately into emergency surgery to close the tear.

Heart Surgery

Cardiac surgery by its very nature is risky. For example, the replacement of a valve, the part of the heart that helps control the direction of blood flow, involves cutting out the diseased valve and suturing in a new one. If the suturing of either the valve or the heart wall is problematic, you could experience bleeding. If the new valve is metal, you may have problems with blood clots. Other complications include heart attack, stroke, even death.

Surgery to Treat Otosclerosis

Otosclerosis is a condition of the middle ear in which the elastic material that surrounds one of the bones becomes inflamed and is converted to bone itself. The material becomes so solid that the bone cannot vibrate and transmit sound, leaving a person deaf. Different surgeries may correct this problem. Most involve substituting another kind of tissue or a metal piston for the troublesome bone to restore hearing. This requires microsurgery. The eardrum is cut and folded back. Then a drill or laser makes a hole for the substitute device. During microsurgery the drill or laser could damage surrounding tissue and bone, or hearing could be compromised if there is a problem reattaching the eardrum.

Craniotomy

Like the heart, the brain is a delicate organ. Because it controls the central nervous system, a complication in some brain surgeries could result in paralysis.

Complications from Anesthesia

Most, though not all, anesthetic complications occur with general anesthesia. In some cases, a patient is unknowingly allergic to the anesthetic. In other cases, the dose is too high or the anesthetic has taken effect faster than desired. Fortunately, numerous other drugs may counteract such adverse reactions. Below is a list of other possible complications.

Airway Obstruction

Some levels of anesthesia may irritate the air passages, causing spasms in the vocal cords and airways and interfering with breathing. If the problem is severe, assisted ventilation will not help. The anesthesiologist may have to insert a tube down the throat or, as a final resort, cut into the windpipe to bypass the problem. With a spinal anesthetic, if the medicine moves higher and temporarily paralyzes your diaphragm, you will also need an incision in your windpipe to restore breathing.

Incomplete Reversal

Muscle relaxants given to render patients immobile during surgery may not completely wear off by the time one regains consciousness. The patient is aware but essentially paralyzed. Fortunately, it is easy to detect the problem, and breathing can be assisted. Sedatives may also be given to calm a patient.

Nerve Damage

Some local anesthetics may cause long-term nerve damage, while some general anesthetics may inflict brain damage. Brain damage may also result from depressed blood circulation. If the body lacks sufficient oxygen for too long, death could occur.

Malignant Hyperthermia (MH)

An uncommon but severe reaction, *MH* results in a dangerous level of hyperactivity of many bodily functions. Body temperature, blood pressure, and heart rate rise to life-threatening extremes. This is a rare complication of general anesthesia that may lead to death if not recognized and treated quickly. A tendency to experience MH may be inherited. If other family members have experienced MH during surgery, alert your surgeon before any operation.

Awareness

Awareness is rare, occurring in 1 percent of surgeries. A patient appears asleep yet is not fully unconscious. If muscle blockers have also been given, the patient cannot move or speak to alert the surgeon. The sensation of pain may or may not be blocked. If a patient has postoperative memories of this experience, he/she often faces psychological problems like insomnia, nightmares, concentration

Medicine and surgery today is more high tech then ever before. I am constantly staying abreast of new developments that will benefit patients. Often, patients ask me about a new technique they've heard about in the news and want to know if they are a candidate for it.

Steve, 39, M.D.
Surgeon

problems, and *post-traumatic stress syndrome*, a psychological reaction occurring after a highly stressful event. This complication occurs from too light a dose of anesthesia.

An observant anesthesiologist might also note certain physical signs, such as increased sweating, tearing, and salivation as well as irregular breathing, spontaneous eye movements, and changes in muscle tone. Newer technology allows anesthesiologists to reliably monitor a patient's sympathetic nervous system, indicating if a patient is awake. Unfortunately, few hospitals have this technology.

Chapter 15

The Recovery Room

After surgery, if you are progressing well and breathing on your own, you will be taken to a recovery room, often called a *post-anesthesia care unit (PACU)*. You may be there for an hour of more, or until you are conscious and your vital signs are stable. Nurses there will constantly monitor and document your blood pressure, heart rate, temperature, and the amount of oxygen in your body. Any unusual changes in these vital signs will be immediately reported to the anesthesiologist or surgeon.

One or more intravenous lines will remain in place so that you may receive a saline solution or other fluids. These will either help rehydrate your body or deliver various medications. You also may have special inflatable stockings on your legs. These are hooked up to a unit that pumps them up periodically. The stockings will help prevent blood clots from forming in your legs. This is particularly important if you won't be mobile very soon after surgery. You will not be allowed any visitors in the recovery room.

Intensive Care Unit

In some cases, patients are taken not to a regular recovery room but instead to an *intensive care unit (ICU)*. There, the ratio of medical and nursing staff to patients is higher. These professionals are specially trained in resuscitation techniques.

Patients typically taken to an ICU after surgery include those who can't breathe on their own and require a ventilator; those who have undergone a major operation like a transplant, heart-bypass, or removal of the colon; those who have been in emergency surgery; those who are seriously ill or have other underlying health problems; and the elderly.

When I woke up in the recovery room after my operation it felt like the room was spinning. I had tubes in me and heard strange noises. The nurses who took care of me were compassionate and explained everything.
Holly, 28
Patient

Possible Side Effects of Anesthesia

Although the surgery may be behind you, it's not uncommon to feel sick while coming out from under general anesthesia. Post-surgical patients report a variety of symptoms as the anesthesia wears off.

Chills

Many patients feel cold and shiver immediately after waking up from surgery. This is caused, in part, by gases from the general anesthetic still in the blood. As the gases dissipate in your bloodstream, you'll feel warmer. Additional factors may be the cool temperature in the operating room and a thin hospital gown. It's also okay to ask for a warm blanket.

Nausea

Although your stomach will be empty, you may feel as if you're going to vomit.

Often called *dry heaves*, this condition may be quite unpleasant.

Irritated Throat or Nasal Passages

You may find that your throat is sore, or you may be hoarse as the result of a breathing tube placed down your windpipe during the operation. This is usually a minor complaint. The soreness should disappear within twenty-four to forty-eight hours. In the meantime, drinking fluids or taking a throat lozenge may bring relief.

Your nasal passages may have been irritated by a nasogastric tube placed through your nose and into your stomach to keep the stomach empty during surgery. Some operations, such as major intestinal or stomach surgery, may require that this tube be kept in place for several days. Many patients find the tube uncomfortable and have a natural tendency to pull it out. Ask your surgeon before the operation whether this tube will be used and whether it will remain postoperatively. Once the tube is taken out, the irritation will subside.

After waking up from surgery, patients can be really disoriented. They can actually hurt themselves by pulling on their tubes or hitting their incision site. My job as a recovery room nurse is to not let this happen by talking to them and reassuring them.

Ron, 40
Recovery Room Nurse

Delayed Ability to Urinate

Another tube that may be inserted before or during your surgery is a *Foley catheter*. This tube runs through the urethra and into the bladder to keep the bladder empty during surgery. It is often removed in the operating room. If your surgeon feels that your muscles will respond sluggishly and that you will be unable to urinate immediately, the Foley catheter may remain in place. How long is up to your surgeon. You should experience no pain from its position once the catheter is inside the bladder, although you may have the sensation of wanting to empty your bladder even when it already is empty.

> *It can be traumatic for a patient's family to see their loved one in the intensive care unit immediately after an operation. I try to lessen that trauma when the family visits by answering their questions and calming their fears.*
>
> *Karen, 38*
> *Intensive Care Nurse*

Headache

You will be more likely to suffer a headache if you've had spinal anesthesia. Spinal fluid may have leaked from the spot where the needle was inserted to administer the anesthetic. The risk is small, but the resulting headache may be severe. If a headache develops, it will likely occur within twenty-four to seventy-two hours after surgery. It may last for several days, until the needle hole heals shut. Drugs may relieve the pain, but the most reliable treatment is an *epidural blood patch*. In this procedure, the anesthesiologist performs another epidural near the site of the first one and injects a small amount of your own blood to form a clot, patching the original hole.

Pain Control

As discussed in an early chapter, you will likely feel pain as anesthesia and muscle relaxants wear off after the operation. To provide the fastest relief possible, your anesthesiologist will likely prescribe an *opioid analgesic* such as morphine. Opioid analgesics have a sedative effect that produce greater comfort.

Chapter 16

Your Hospital Room

Once you leave the recovery room or an intensive care unit, you'll be moved to a regular hospital room, where your recuperation will continue. Don't be surprised if the hospital staff has you out of bed and moving soon after surgery. In fact, many cardiovascular patients will be helped up and around even while they are still recovering in an intensive care unit. Although taking those first steps may be painful, getting back on your feet is important. Movement helps prevent pneumonia (caused by fluids settling in the lungs), improve circulation, reduce the chance of blood clots, and strengthen the muscles.

If your surgery involved orthopedic surgery from the hips down, however, walking will be discouraged at first to allow you to heal. A patient recovering from abdominal surgery will often get support, typically a pillow, to place over the incision. The pillow will take some of the pressure off the incision. Since you may initially feel weak or dizzy, at least one nurse or aide will help you walk.

The Hospital Room

How hospital rooms are equipped varies, depending on the needs of patients. Private rooms are available, but most are semiprivate, meaning they are set up for two patients. Some hospitals may have larger rooms for four people or more. Many insurance plans will not pay for private rooms.

Roommates

If you're in a semiprivate room, you most likely will have a roommate. Often, having a roommate is a pleasant experience, bringing you companionship during your hospital stay. Other times, you and the roommate may not be well suited to share a room. If this should be the case, talk to your nurses about your options for moving to a different room. If you are in a semiprivate room, you'll want to be considerate of your roommate's privacy and, in turn, expect the same respect from your roommate. Many hospitals have lounges where you and your visitors may wish to visit.

Beds

Most patients will have a typical hospital bed—a single bed that may be raised or lowered at the head and feet. Controls for adjusting the bed will normally be placed on the guard-rails. These rails may be raised for patients at risk of falling out of bed.

Some rooms will have specialty beds, depending on the needs of the patients. For patients who are bedfast for extended periods of time, skin breakdown, or *bedsores*, may occur. To prevent this, special beds with mattresses that inflate and deflate are available. These special mattresses prevent a single point of constant pressure on patients. Other beds have special air mattresses or gelatinous substances that provide motion. There are even beds that use shifting sand to eliminate pressure.

Another type of specialty bed features a striker frame, which holds two stretcher beds. These "sandwich" a patient, permitting him/her to be turned without being touched. This type of bed also may be used for patients whose conditions make them difficult to turn, including paraplegics, quadriplegics, or the very obese.

Intercom

The intercom system, or buzzer, in your room connects you to the nursing station. If you need help, you should be able to press your buzzer and receive a response. A nurse or an aide will come to your room as soon as possible. If the staff is busy with other patients, it may take a few minutes for them to arrive.

Bathroom

Most hospital rooms will include a bathroom complete with a toilet, hand sink, and mirror. Some bathrooms will also have showers or bathtubs. If not, you may be taken to a nearby room where a shower or bathtub is available. If you are unable to walk to the bathroom to use the toilet, you may need to use a bedpan or bedside commode. It is normal to feel initial embarrassment about using one. Keep in mind that hospital staff are very used to patients using bedpans and bedside commodes. They treat it simply as part of your recovery.

Amenities

Most hospital rooms will have at least one television, and there usually is a clock. Many rooms suspend a small television above the head of the bed for private viewing. If you have a roommate, then you will probably have to work out a viewing schedule. If you want to bring in any other electronic equipment, first ask for permission from the hospital staff. Many items like cellular phones and even computers may emit signals that distort the hospital's electronic monitoring systems.

Each room usually has a telephone. The more recent trend is for each bed to have a telephone. The telephone is tied to a central switchboard. In most hospitals, the operators will switch off all patients' telephones at a certain time. Ask about the policy for incoming calls. Keep in mind that, for privacy reasons, many hospitals will not let a caller know that you are a patient in the hospital.

Hospital Routines & Schedules

While every hospital has its own routines, most have similar methods of operation. They are in operation twenty-four hours a day, seven days a week, and are staffed by dozens to hundreds of people. Personnel shifts for most health care workers (excluding physicians) typically run from 7:00 A.M. to 3:00 P.M., 3:00 P.M. to 11:00 P.M., and 11:00 P.M. to 7:00 A.M. Some hospitals run two twelve-hour shifts, 7:00 A.M. to 7:00 P.M. and 7:00 P.M. to 7:00 A.M.

I play a role in the discharge planning of many surgical patients. I try to answer questions regarding what to expect at home once discharged. Often, patients and their families remember questions once the surgeon leaves the room so they ask me.

Karen, 38
Ward Nurse

Physician Visits

You will usually be seen by a doctor at least once a day during the time he/she makes "rounds," the period during which physicians make regular checks on patients. At times, you may be visited by your surgeon. At other times, you may be seen by your primary care physician. If you are with an HMO or similar type of plan, the physician attending at the hospital that day may visit you. During these visits, your physician will check your chart, ask how you're feeling, examine you, and review your medications.

Nurse and Therapist Visits

You will be visited by members of the nursing staff frequently. Depending on the management of the hospital, you may be assigned to a primary nurse during the day and at other times to associate nurses. During your first two to four days in the hospital, a nurse or aide will stop by every four to six hours to check your blood pressure, pulse, and temperature.

If you require therapy, a therapist will visit you early on to assess your condition. Depending on your mobility, your therapy will take place either in your room or in the hospital's therapy clinic. Most respiratory therapy is done bedside.

Delivery of Medication

Typically medications are given around 5:00 A.M., 11:00 A.M., 5:00 P.M., and 11:00 P.M. Nurses will arrive within a half hour of that time with your medication. Some medication may be given through your IV line. Other medicine may be given by injection, often referred to as *IM*, or intramuscular. Still other times, you may receive a pill.

Meals

Most hospitals serve three meals a day. Breakfast is usually served around 7:00 A.M., lunch between 11:30 A.M. and 12:30 P.M., and dinner between 5:30 and 6:30 P.M. Some hospitals will circulate a menu several hours before mealtimes, offering you a choice. All menus are planned by dietitians, who ensure that meals are balanced and nutritious.

Your diet may be restricted, depending on the kind of surgery you had. For example, if you've had gastrointestinal surgery, you may require light, soft meals that are easily digested.

Visitors

Now that you're in a regular hospital room, family and friends may visit. Most hospitals have visitation guidelines, restricting the number of people who may visit you at one time. Many hospitals also do not permit visitors under the age of twelve. All these guidelines are to your benefit. Too many visitors may be stressful and tiring while you are recuperating.

Chapter 17

Leaving the Hospital

B efore your operation, you probably discussed with your doctor how much time you would spend in the hospital. Most surgeons should be able to provide a reasonable time estimate based on the type of surgery. Insurance companies also are interested in these estimates, and often grant approval to cover you for only a certain number of days. If the estimate your surgeon provides and the number of approved days are different, you may wish to call your insurance company to discuss what happens if you must stay longer.

Estimated Length of Hospital Stays

A surgeon will sign your discharge papers when you are ready to leave the hospital. If your surgery turns out to be more complicated than originally thought, you may have to stay longer. For example, if an infection sets in, you probably won't be released until the infection is under control. On the other hand, if your in-hospital recovery goes better than expected, you may be able to leave early.

Before you are dismissed, your health care team also will want to confirm that your bodily functions are returning to normal. It's important that your bowels and kidneys are functioning. Anesthesia and other drugs slow your organs, including the intestines and bladder. Your release also will depend on the results of tests performed in the hospital. The results will tell your surgeon if your recovery is on track and if you are responding correctly to medications.

Operations & Average Days in Hospital			
Repair an aneurysm	5-10	Cardiac bypass grafting	5-10
Carotid endarterectomy	2-4	Implant a pacemaker	1-2
Colectomy	5-7	Appendectomy	2-3
Major repair of joints	5-7	Laminectomy/diskectomy	1-3
Fractures requiring open hip surgery	7-10	Fractures requiring open ankle surgery	2-5
Arthroplasty	5-10	Skin graft	5-10
Prostatectomy	5-7	Hysterectomy	2-5
Mastectomy	1-3	Pulmonary resection	4-10
Craniotomy	5-10		

Questions for Your Nurses and Doctors

Before you leave the hospital, you will probably be visited by your doctor, who will discuss your operation. Since you may still be dealing with the effects of your surgery or medications, you may not remember to find out all the information you'll want later. Your doctor's answers to the following questions will be helpful.

- How would you describe the results of the operation?
- What exactly did you find?
- Did the surgery take longer than normal?

- Were there any complications? Will those complications affect my recuperation at home?
- How should I expect my recovery to progress?
- Will I need treatment from another physician or specialist?

It is important to thoroughly understand the results of your operation. Don't be afraid or embarrassed to ask your surgeon to explain things to you more than once if you don't understand. This is especially true if the news after your surgery isn't as hopeful as you would have liked. For example, if you were having lymph nodes removed because you were diagnosed with cancer, and your surgeon found that tumors had spread, you would want as much information as possible.

We try to prepare patients with special needs, such as a colostomy or an open wound, on what to expect at home. Patients are very anxious when they get home, especially if they need special care. Maintaining an open line of communication is crucial to comforting patients during their recovery.
Sonya, 35
Home Health Nurse

When you are ready to leave the hospital, you probably will have at least one nurse discuss do's and don'ts for your recuperation. The hospital will have discharge papers for you to sign that will contain information about your continuing care. But these papers may have only the simplest instructions. Your surgeon's office may provide more printed materials for you as well. Again, make sure you understand *everything* before you leave. Arrange time to talk with a nurse and anyone else you feel should provide input about your recuperation.

In an earlier chapter, questions to ask about your recovery were listed; however, you may wish to refer to the following list to make sure you have all the information you need.

- When should I schedule a follow-up appointment with my surgeon?
- Will I need assistance from a trained aide at home?
- Should I continue my current medication(s)?
- Will I need any special medications, antibiotics, or pain pills? For how long?
- How long will I experience discomfort?
- When do the bandages come off?
- How should I care for my incision?
- Will any stitches or staples be removed? When?
- When may I shower or bathe again?
- Is it okay to lift things? Up to how much weight?
- When may I drive again?
- When may I return to a normal diet?
- What complications may arise after I go home?
- When should I call the doctor if I'm concerned about my condition?

> *I tell patients and their families if any questions arise at home feel free to call my office. Someone will be there to help.*
>
> *Dan, M.D.*
> *Surgeon*

As you ask questions, don't hesitate to take notes. Do not rely solely on your memory. You may ask a family member or friend to take notes for you.

If you will need assistance from a home-health nurse or aide, make sure this has been requested and approved. That request will probably have to come from your surgeon's office and be approved by your insurance company. When you finally leave the

---

Discharge Checklist

- Surgeon's office number and date of follow-up appointment (if already made)
- Surgeon's answering service number
- Names of surgeon's partners
- Instructions for care of wound(s)
- Warning signs or problems (excessive pain, infection, vomiting, fever)
- Special instructions for activity level, diet, showering, driving, walking, exercising, returning to work, resuming sexual relations
- Prescriptions
- Insurance paperwork

---

hospital, make sure that you have all the items noted in the discharge checklist above.

Medications at Discharge

Now that it is time to leave the hospital, you may receive prescriptions for additional medications. You will most likely be given a prescription for a pain medication. Whether you need it is a question only you can answer.

Upon discharge, some patients also receive a card stating that they have a pacemaker, heart defibrillator, plastic patches or supports, pins, or an indwelling catheter. If you have an item that may set off airport and other security systems, the card will explain it. Always carry the card with you, since you never know when you may need it.

What If I Need Additional Care?

Some patients leaving the hospital may need additional, specialized care. This is especially true of patients who need rehabilitation. They may go to a rehabilitation center before going home. Additionally, patients who will need assistance, but do not have family members or others to provide that help, might consider an assisted-care facility.

Still other patients may face leaving the hospital in the final stages of a terminal disease that surgery could not slow or arrest. These patients and their families must decide whether to return home or transfer to another care facility, such as a hospice.

When you do finally leave the hospital, you will be expected to have transportation, unless you are being transferred to another location via ambulance. As you leave the hospital ward, you will not be allowed to walk to the exit, but will be taken in a wheelchair. You may have to stop at the billing office first to answer questions, but not necessarily to pay your bill at this time.

Chapter 18

Recovering at Home

Your surgery and time in the hospital are over. It's time to return home. Just walking through the door into that familiar environment should boost your morale. Hopefully, your support system—family, friends, even pets—will aid your continued recovery.

What to Expect

When you first arrive home, you will likely still feel some pain or fatigue. The following symptoms are normal during recovery at home:

- Pain, discomfort, and/or a pulling sensation that are relieved by pain medication and do not increase in intensity
- Minor bleeding or drainage stain covering a small portion of the bandage
- Redness (develops in about a week) around staples or sutures only, meaning it is time for them to be removed
- Diminished appetite
- Fatigue

When to Call the Doctor

However, some problems at home demand immediate attention. If you notice any of the following warning signs, call your physician or emergency services immediately.

- A fever of 101° F. or higher occurring within the first twenty-four to forty-eight hours after surgery
- Substantial or constant nausea or vomiting
- Lightheadedness, dizziness
- Shortness of breath
- Unusual/excessive bleeding or bruising
- Signs of infection at your incision, including swelling, redness, warmth, pain, or drainage, particularly if it has an odor
- Pain that medication does not relieve
- Pain beyond the incision site that keeps getting worse, such as chest pain that spreads to the jaw or arm

Levels of Care

The level of care you will need after surgery is something you and your surgeon should discuss before the operation. Most patients will be able to handle most routines once they get home.

In some cases, you will need assistance. A family member or friend may be able to help you with everyday activities like grooming and meal preparation.

After I went home from my heart surgery, I had been told what to expect, but I was still scared and called my doctor several times during my recovery. Each time, the nurses in his office were understanding and very helpful in getting me through my recovery.

John, 67
Patient

Or, you may need further help, at least when you first get home. For example, you may not be able to walk without assistance. In this case, you may require the services of a home-health aide. You will need to speak with your surgeon's office about this, or the hospital's discharge planner may be able to schedule an aide for you. If you are with an HMO, you may first need to contact, or have your nurse or surgeon contact, the appropriate department in your organization to make those arrangements.

Still others will need another category of care. For instance, a nurse may be needed to give injections, dress wounds, and check vital signs such as pulse and respiration. You may need visits from a home-health nurse. They visit patients in their homes to provide whatever medical assistance is needed. You may also require the services of other health care professionals. Perhaps you were sent home with oxygen and need respiratory therapy. Or perhaps you need to relearn daily activities and require occupational therapy but are in no shape to travel outside your home.

Physical Activity and Diet

Physical activity and nutrition are two significant factors in your recovery. Physical activity ranges from just getting out of bed in the morning to taking progressively longer walks to having intensive physical-therapy sessions. Physical exercise is important to your cardiovascular health. Exercise keeps your blood circulating normally. If you are too inactive, your circulation may become sluggish, increasing the risk of blood clots forming in the slow-moving blood. These clots may cause serious problems, including stroke or heart attack.

If physical therapy is prescribed, a physical therapist will help you with a series of exercises designed specifically to strengthen your muscles and regain stamina. You may need to begin some sessions at home, then progress to a rehabilitation program at a different center or hospital. In some cases, your physical therapy may take place in a swimming pool because it has been shown that exercising in water is gentler on the body's joints. Wherever you perform physical therapy, the goal is the same: to get you back on your feet.

The importance of good nutrition cannot be understated. An appropriate diet may help speed your recovery, while a poor diet may compromise it. As a result of your surgery, you need to make dietary changes. If you have been diagnosed with a heart problem, for example, a healthy diet will be very important. As you may realize, heart disease is often caused by a poor diet high in fats that allows plaque to build up in the arteries. Accordingly, you may be given dietary instructions that call for more fruits, vegetables, and grains, and less fats and sugars. If you have high blood pressure, the sodium in your diet will likely be restricted. If you have problems with gastric acid, you may be put on a diet that prohibits spicy foods.

During the follow-up office visit, my surgeon told me a lot of my complaints recovering at home were normal for the operation I had. I had no idea this was the case. He also told me about the pathology report on the gallbladder he removed; I never would have thought to ask.

Danielle, 27
Patient

Emotional Ups and Downs

Just as your physical health is important, so is your mental health. You have just been through a physically traumatic experience that may also have impacted your emotional well-being. For most people, anticipating surgery is stressful and tense, mixed with the feeling that the operation will help resolve certain physical problems. Post-operatively, you might expect that recovery will be a very positive experience. For many people it is.

However, for many others, the period after surgery is one of depression and increased anxiety. It is not uncommon to experience a postsurgical letdown. Why? Patients may think they're not recovering as fast as they should. Perhaps they've heard about relatives who were up and around in two days after having the same surgery. Other patients may find the pain is worse than expected, or learn they can't go back to work as soon as expected. Still others may fear they'll never regain their health. All of these beliefs may lead one to withdraw and sink into depression.

Many patients come back to my office with questions about their operation, their incision, and what to expect before getting back to normal. Most of the time patients are relieved to find out what they are experiencing is just part of the healing process.

Steve, 39, M.D.
Surgeon

The problem could also result from a chemical imbalance in the body, particularly if you're taking new medications or have had hormonal changes as a result of the surgery. Pay close attention to how you are reacting mentally and physically to any new medications. If you suspect something is wrong, talk to your physician. It could be that switching medications will relieve your depression.

If family members or friends tell you that you seem depressed, listen carefully to what they are saying. You are not necessarily in the best position to assess your mood, but someone who observes you a great deal during the day and knows how you act normally is. This is a time to accept support. If family members or friends suggest you call your doctor—or do it themselves—understand that they act out of love and concern for you. You may need to talk to a counselor, or taking antidepressants may help.

Any number of life's simple pleasures may lift one's spirits: a good book, a movie, sunshine cascading into your room, the love of a pet. Studies show that a human-animal bond may actually lower a person's blood pressure, stress level, and heart rate while increasing one's emotional well-being. Your pet provides unconditional love. When you're feeling low, this love is emotionally nourishing.

Follow-Up Appointment

During your follow-up appointment with your doctor or surgeon, you will be examined to determine how well you're healing from surgery. The dressing over your incision will probably be changed or removed. If the operation limited your mobility, your surgeon will likely have you go through some movements to see whether your range of motion is improving. Anything related to how you are progressing will be covered.

It's likely that your stitches will be removed during this visit. Many stitches or sutures used today are absorbable and need not be removed. Nonabsorbable stitches or staples are usually removed five to ten days after surgery. Other stitches may be internal. You'll never see them. They will dissolve. Any exposed suture knots from the internal stitches will eventually drop off on their own.

Stitches are removed with scissors or a special scalpel. You shouldn't feel any pain as they're removed. However, you might feel a slight tugging as a suture is pulled out. Sometimes they stick to each other or to body hairs. If this happens, a nurse or doctor may soak them in a saline solution to free them before snipping. To remove staples or skin clips, the surgeon uses a device that resembles a small pair of pliers. It bends the staple or skin clip so that the ends separate.

Future Follow-Up or Treatment

For many patients, a single follow-up appointment is enough. If all is progressing well, you may be discharged from your surgeon's care. Or, you may be referred to specialists for additional treatment. For example, you may start seeing a cardiologist regularly if your surgery involved your heart. Individuals who had a cancerous tumor removed may undergo chemotherapy, radiation therapy, or some combination of both. If your surgery involved joints in your arms, legs, or back, then you will likely be scheduled for physical therapy to help rebuild your strength.

Your recovery will rely in large part on how well you follow your prescribed activities after the operation. The more you comply, the speedier your recovery. The goal is to heal and return to a normal life as quickly and completely as possible.

Resources

Consumer-Oriented Associations

American Cancer Society
1599 Clifton Road NE
Atlanta, GA 30329-4251
1-800-ACS-2345 (1-800-227-2345)
www.cancer.org

American Diabetes Association
1701 North Beauregard Street
Alexandria, VA 22311
1-800-DIABETES (1-800-342-2383)
www.diabetes.org

American Heart Association
(National Center mailing address)
National Center
7272 Greenville Avenue
Dallas, Texas 75231
   Consumer Heart and Stroke Information
   1-800-AHA-USA1 (1-800-242-8721)
   Women's Health Information
   1-888-MY-HEART (1-800-694-3278)
www.amhrt.org

Brain Injury Association, Inc.
105 North Alfred Street
Alexandria, VA 22314
Phone: 703-236-6000
Fax: 703-236-6001
www.biausa.org

National Kidney Foundation
30 East 33rd Street
Suite 1100
New York, NY 10016
Phone: 1-800-622-9010
212-889-2210
Fax: 212-689-9261
www.kidney.org

National Stroke Association
96 Inverness Drive East
Suite I
Englewood, CO 80112-5112
Phone: 303.649.9299
Fax: 303.649.1328
1-800-STROKES (1-800-787-6537)
www.stroke.org

Y-ME National Breast Cancer Organization
212 West Van Buren Street
Chicago, IL 60607-3908
24-hour toll-free hotlines:
1-800-221-2141 ENGLISH
1-800-986-9505 SPANISH
www.y-me.org

Physician Organizations

American Academy of Pain Medicine
700 West Lake Avenue
Glenville, IL 60025
Phone: 708-966-9510
Fax: 708-375-4777
www.painmed.org

American College of Gastroenterology

4900-B South 31st Street
Arlington, VA 22206
Phone: 703-820-7400
Fax: 703-931-4520
www.acg.gi.org

American College of Obstetricians and Gynecologists

409 12th Street, South West
P.O. Box 96920
Washington, D.C. 20090-6920
202-638-5577
http://www.acog.org

American College of Surgeons

633 North Saint Clair Street
Chicago, IL 60611-3211
312-202-5000
Fax: 312-202-5001
www.facs.org

American Gastroenterological Association

7910 Woodmont Avenue
7th Floor
Bethesda, MD 20814
Phone: 301-654-2055
Fax: 301-654-5920
www.gastro.org

American Medical Association

Headquarters
515 North State Street
Chicago, IL 60610
312-464-5000
www.amuro.org

Washington, D.C. Office
1101 Vermont Avenue NW
Washington, D.C. 20005
202-789-7400
www.ama-assn.org

American Society of Hypertension

515 Madison Avenue
New York, NY 10022
Phone: 212-644-0650
Fax: 212-644-0658
www.ash-us.org

American Urological Association

Headquarters
1120 North Charles Street
Baltimore, MD 21201
Phone: 410-727-1100
Fax: 410-223-4370

Office of Education

2425 West Loop South
Suite 333
Houston, TX 77027-4207
Phone: 1-800-282-7077 or 713-622-2700
Fax: 713-622-2898
www.auanet.org

American Hospital Association

    Headquarters
    One North Franklin
    Chicago, Illinois 60606
    Phone: 312-422-3000
    Fax: 312-422-4796
    http://www.aha.org

    Washington, D.C. Office
    325 Seventh Street North West
    Washington, D.C. 20004
    Phone: 1-800-424-4301 or 202-638-1100
    Fax: 202-626-2345
    www.aha.org

Internet Resources

National Institutes of Health

Comprised of 25 separate institutes and centers, the NIH is one of 8 health agencies in the U.S. Department of Health and Human Services.

National Cancer Institute

National Institutes of Health
Bethesda, MD 20892
301-496-4000
1-800-4-CANCER (1-800-422-6237)
www.nci.nih.gov

National Eye Institute

National Institutes of Health
2020 Vision Place
Bethesda, MD 20892-3655
(301) 496-5248
www.nei.nih.gov

National Heart, Lung & Blood Institute
National Institutes of Health
Bethesda, MD 20892
www.nhlbi.nih.gov

National Institute of Dental & Craniofacial Research
National Institutes of Health
Bethesda, MD 20892
www.nidr.nih.gov

National Institute of Diabetes and Digestive and Kidney Diseases
National Institutes of Health
Bethesda, MD 20892
www.niddk.nih.gov/index.htm

National Center for Complementary and Alternative Medicine
National Institutes of Health
Bethesda, MD 20892
http://nccam.nih.gov/

U.S. Food and Drug Administration
FDA (HFE-88)
5600 Fishers Lane
Rockville, MD 20857
1-888-INFO-FDA (1-888-463-6332)
www.fda.gov
Information about medications.

U.S. Department of Health and Human Services
200 Independence Avenue, S.W.
Washington, D.C. 20201
1-877-696-6775 or 202-619-0257
www.os.dhhs.gov

Healthfinder
www.healthfinder.gov
Consumer information from the U.S. Department of Health and
Human Services.

Agency for Health Care Policy and Research (AHCPR)
2021 K St. NW
Washington, D.C. 20006
202-296-6922
800-358-9295
www.ahcpr.gov

Centers for Disease Control and Prevention
1600 Clifton Road
Atlanta, GA 30333
404-639-3311
www.cdc.gov
Statistics and other information about diseases and conditions.

U.S. National Library of Medicine
8600 Rockville Pike
Bethesda, MD 20894
www.nlm.nih.gov
MEDLINE http://www.nih.gov
Produced by the National Library of Medicine, this site indexes
articles from more than 3,500 medical journals. The service is
aimed primarily at scientists and health professionals.

MEDLINEplus http://www.nlm.nih.gov/medlineplus

National Library of Medicine Resources
National Cancer Institute
National Eye Institute
National Heart, Lung, and Blood Institute
National Human Genome Research Institute
National Institute of Arthritis and Musculoskeletal and Skin
    Diseases
National Institute of Child Health and Human Development
National Institute of Dental and Craniofacial Research
National Institute of Diabetes and Digestive and Kidney Diseases
National Institute of Mental Health
National Institute of Neurological Disorders and Stroke
National Institute on Aging
National Institute on Alcohol Abuse and Alcoholism
National Institute on Deafness and Other Communication
    Disorders
National Institutes of Health
National Institutes of Health, Office of Research on Women's
    Health
National Library of Medicine
Agency for Health-care Policy and Research
Centers for Disease Control and Prevention
Environmental Protection Agency
Food and Drug Administration
Health-care Financing Administration
National Institute on Disability and Rehabilitation Research
Office of Disease Prevention and Health Promotion
Alliance of Genetic Support Groups
Alzheimer's Association
American Academy of Dermatology
American Academy of Family Physicians
American Academy of Pediatrics
American Cancer Society
American Chiropractic Association
American College of Gastroenterology

American College of Rheumatology
American Dental Association
American Diabetes Association
American Dietetic Association
American Heart Association
American Hospital Association
American Lung Association
American Medical Association
American Osteopathic Association
American Pharmaceutical Association
American Psychiatric Association
American Psychological Association
American Public Health Association
American Red Cross
American Society of Anesthesiologists
American Veterinary Medical Association
Association for Health Services Research
Association of American Medical Colleges
Federation of State Medical Boards of the United States
Leukemia Society of America
Pan American Health Organization
World Health Organization

More Consumer Health Sites on the Internet

Mayo Clinic Health Oasis www.mayohealth.org
> Mayo Clinic site includes disease and condition reports, health news and features, Ask a Physician, library, and glossary.

InteliHealth www.intelihealth.com
> Johns Hopkins health information center features news and special reports, disease and condition guide, live chat, medical dictionary, physician locator, drug resource center, and newsletter.

AMA Physician Select www.ama-assn.org
From the American Medical Association, this site provides information on nearly every licensed physician in the United States.

HospitalSelect www.hospitalselect.com
A hospital locator, providing information on virtually every hospital in the United States provided in cooperation with the American Medical Association.

Healthgrades www.healthgrades.com
Profiles more than 500,000 hospitals and 600,000 physicians.

Medical Journals on Yahoo http://dir.yahoo.com/Health/
Medicine/Journals
Links to numerous medical journals.

4Cancer.com www.ca.cancer.org
From the American Cancer Society, this site features information on types of cancer, prevention, treatments, research, statistics, and links to other sites.

OBGYN.Net www.obgyn.net/home.htm
A physician-reviewed service, offering information on obstetrics and gynecology for consumers and medical professionals.

American Pain Society www.ampainsoc.org
More than 3,200 doctors, nurses, scientists, psychologists, and pharmacologists who research and treat pain and act as advocates for patients in pain.

Mayday Pain Resource Center http://mayday.coh.org
Pain resource center by City of Hope Medical Center, Duarte, CA.

HealthNewsDigest.com
News on health, science, technology, and the environment.

WebMD www.webMD.com
General health information. Features live chats with experts.

drkoop.com www.drkoop.com

Site by Dr. Everett Koop, former surgeon general. Features health news, resources, reports on health conditions, and insurance information.

Mediconsult.com www.Mediconsult.com

Comprehensive information on health conditions, live chat with experts, message boards.

DiscoveryHealth.com www.discoveryhealth.com

Reports on health for men, women, seniors, and children; health at work; nutrition; fitness; and weight control.

AccentHealth.com www.accenthealth.com

Information on men's, women's, and children's health; drugs; nutrition. Features message boards, comprehensive list of medical tests and procedures.

allHealth.com www.allHealth.com

Part of the *i*Village network for women, this site offers reports on health conditions, wellness and diet, news and special reports, drug data base, chats with experts, message boards.

Glossary

A

Abscess: Collection of pus.

Abdominal aortic aneurysm (AAA): Dilation of the major artery in the abdominal cavity.

Abdominal cavity: Space between the diaphragm and the pelvis that houses major internal organs.

Advance directive: Legal document addressing the use of life support measures if required.

American Board of Surgery: Governing surgical society that oversees surgeons in the United States.

Analgesic: A substance that relieves pain.

Anesthesiologist: A physician who specializes in the administration of anesthesia.

Aneurysm: Abnormal dilation of any blood vessel in the body.

Angiography: The injection of x-ray dye into blood vessels.

Angioplasty: Technique of opening arteries with a balloon.

Anus: Lower opening of the gastrointestinal tract involved in defecation.

Asphyxiation pneumonia: An infection in the lungs caused by the aspiration of stomach contents.

Augmentation: Enlargement, as in breast augmentation.

Appendix: Worm-shaped organ at the junction of the small and large intestines.

Appendectomy: Surgical removal of the appendix.

Arrhythmia: Irregular heartbeat.

Artery: Blood vessel that carries oxygenated blood to the body.

Arthroscope: Long, thin fiber-optic camera used by orthopedic surgeons during surgery.

Arthroscopic surgery: Surgical procedures using an arthroscope.

Aspiration: The act of stomach contents inadvertently entering the lungs.

Asthma: Disease of the passageways in the lungs that causes them to go into spasm.

Atrial fibrillation: Rapid, irregular beating of the upper chamber of the heart.

Audiologist: An individual trained in testing and evaluating hearing.

Autologous blood donation: The act of setting aside your own blood several weeks prior to surgery in anticipation of requiring a transfusion.

B

Bedsore: Trauma to skin and underlying tissues caused by an inability to move.

Benign: Not cancerous or malignant.

Bile duct: Pipelike structure that carries bile from the liver to the intestine.

Biopsy: Surgical removal of a portion or all of a mass or organ.

Bladder: Organ that collects urine from the kidneys.

Bronchitis: Infection of the tubelike passageways in the lungs.

C

Cardiac catheterization: Technique of placing a catheter into the chambers of the heart and injecting dye into the arteries of the heart.

Cardiologist: Physician who specializes in diseases of the heart.

Cardiopulmonary: Related to the heart and lungs.

Cardiothoracic: Related to the heart and organs of the chest cavity.

Cardiovascular technologist: Health care worker trained in assisting a cardiologist perform tests on the heart.

Carpal tunnel syndrome: Disease causing numbness and weakness in the fingers due to nerve compression in the wrist.

Cartilage: Connective tissue in the body found in joints and organs.

Carotid Artery: Main arteries in the neck that carry blood to the brain.

Carotid endarterectomy: Surgical removal of plaque from the carotid artery.

Cataract: Disease of the lens of the eye causing decreased vision.

Cautery: Heating device used to stop bleeding in the operating room.

Cesarean section: Surgical delivery of a newborn.

Cervix: Lower part of the uterus that opens into the vagina.

Cholecystectomy: Surgical removal of the gallbladder.

Chronic obstructive pulmonary disease (COPD): Disease affecting the air passages of the lungs.

Circulating nurse: A nurse who "circulates" in and out of the operating room, retrieving supplies and instruments for the surgeon.

Coronary artery: Main blood vessel supplying the heart with oxygenated blood.

Coronary artery bypass grafting (CABG): Surgically rerouting the blood supply around a blockage in the coronary artery.

Colectomy: Surgical removal of part or all of the colon.

Colon: Large intestine.

Colonoscopy: Procedure to examine the colon with a fiber-optic scope.

Computerized axial tomography (CAT Scan): Special x-ray technique to evaluate organs and tissues in the body.

Contrast media: Liquid or dye injected or swallowed which illuminates organs and tissues during x-ray tests.

Craniotomy: Operation removing a piece of skull to gain access to the brain.

Cyst: Noncancerous growth, usually filled with fluid.

Cystectomy: Operation to remove part or all of the bladder.

D

Defibrillator: Electrical device used to shock the heart into a normal beat.

Diabetes: Disease affecting the cells of the pancreas, which controls blood sugars.

Dietician: Health care worker trained to consult patients regarding daily food intake and diet.

Disk: Structures supporting the bony skeleton of the spinal column.

Discectomy: Removal of part or all of a vertebral disk.

Diverticulosis: Disease that causes small weak spots and outpouchings in the colon wall.

Diverticulitis: Disease that occurs when outpouchings in the colon wall become infected.

Doppler ultrasound: X-ray test using sound waves to evaluate tissues and organs.

Dry heaves: The action of vomiting without stomach contents coming up.

Durable Health Care Power of Attorney (Health Care Proxy): Legal directive, designating another as a decision-maker should the patient become incapable.

E

Echocardiogram: Diagnostic test using ultrasound to evaluate heart valves and heart function.

Electrocardiogram: A static tracing of the heart's rhythm.

Electroencephalogram (EEG): Dynamic tracing of the activity of the brain.

Emphysema: Disease that results in the destruction of normal lung tissue.

Endoscopy: Procedure that looks into the esophagus and stomach with a fiber-optic scope.

ENT (Ear, Nose, and Throat): A physician who specializes in diseases of the head, ear, nose, throat, and neck. Also known as an otolaryngologist.

Enzyme: A specialized protein that acts as a catalyst during chemical reactions in the body.

Epidural: Anesthetic method in which medicine is injected around the lining of the spinal column.

Epidural blood patch: Technique used to treat headaches that occur after spinal anesthesia.

Epilepsy: Neurological disease of the brain that results in seizures.

Esophagus: Tube through which food passes from the mouth to the stomach.

Esophagectomy: Surgical removal of all or part of the esophagus.

Estrogen: Female hormone.

F

Fallopian tubes: Organs that connect the ovaries to the uterus for the passage of eggs.

Fellowship: Advanced training for surgeons to become specialists.

Foley Catheter: Plastic tube inserted through the urethra and into the bladder to empty the bladder.

Fracture: A break, as in a broken bone.

G

Gag reflex: Involuntary reflex causing gagging by contact with the back of the throat.

130

Gallbladder: Organ under the liver that stores bile, involved in the digestion of fatty foods.

Gastric: Related to the stomach.

General anesthesia: Anesthesia used during surgery causing the patient to be asleep.

Gurney: Bed on wheels used to transport patients within the hospital.

Gynecologist: Physician specializing in treating female disorders and delivering newborns.

H

Hammertoe: Diseased bones in a toe that causes pain and deformity.

Hemoglobin: Complex molecule in red blood cells that transports oxygen to tissues.

Hemorrhoids: Abnormal veins around the anus that cause pain and bleeding.

Hemorrhoidectomy: Surgical removal of hemorrhoids.

Hernia: Weakness or defect in tissues, commonly seen in the groin.

Herniated: Weakened or bulging, such as a disc in the spinal column compressing on nerves.

Home-health aide: Health care worker who assists patients at home with basic needs.

Home-health nurse: Nurse who specializes in assisting patients at home during recovery.

Homocysteine: An amino acid found in the body. Abnormally high levels are associated with an increased risk of heart disease.

Hysterectomy: Surgical removal of the uterus.

I

Infarction: Blockage of blood supply and oxygen, which causes cells to die.

Insulin: Substance made by the pancreas that controls sugar levels in the blood.

Intensive Care Unit-ICU: Hospital area where acutely ill patients go to recover after major surgery.

Internship: Name given to the first year of training for surgeons just out of medical school.

Intramuscular (IM): Referring to inside a muscle, as in giving an injection.

Intravenous line (IV): A thin, hollow tube placed inside an arm vein to administer fluids or drugs intravenously.

J – K

Joint Commission for Accreditation of Healthcare Organizations (JCAHO): Governing body that overlooks and inspects hospitals.

L

Laminectomy: Surgical removal of excess bone in the spinal column.

Laparoscope: Fiber-optic tube connected to a TV monitor, used during surgery.

Laparoscopic surgery: Surgery using the laparoscope to visualize organs.

Larynx: Structure in the throat that houses the vocal cords.

Licensed Practical Nurse (LPN): A nurse assistant who has one year of training and has passed a state test to receive a license.

Ligaments: Fibrous bands that hold bones and joints together.

Liposuction: Surgical procedure to remove excess fat.

Living will: Document explaining a patient's wishes for the use of life support measures in case he/she is incapacitated.

Lobectomy: Surgical removal of part of a lung.

Local anesthesia: Injection of medicine into an area, numbing it to pain so a surgeon can perform local surgery.

Lymph nodes: Structures throughout the body that fight infections.

M

Magnetic Resonance Imaging (MRI): Highly specialized x-ray using electrons to take detailed pictures of organs and tissues.

Major surgery: Surgery involving major organ systems, requiring general anesthesia, and prolonged hospital stay.

Malignant: Tending to produce death or deterioration.

Malignant hyperthermia: Uncommon disease brought on by general anesthesia resulting in potential fever, heart failure, kidney failure, and possible death.

Mastectomy: Surgical removal of a breast.

Membrane: A layer of tissue surrounding an organ or other structure.

Menopause: Natural cessation of the menstrual cycle.

Microsurgery: Surgery on fine structures using magnified glasses or a microscope.

Minimally Invasive Surgery: Surgery using smaller instruments and incisions.

Minor surgery: Surgery requiring any type of anesthesia, performed as an outpatient or in a doctor's office, and resulting in a short recovery time.

Myocardial: Referring to the heart.

Myocardial Infarction (MI): Heart attack, or blockage of blood to the heart.

N

Narcotic: Potent drug given to treat pain after surgery.

Nasogastric tube: Tube inserted in the nose to empty the stomach.

Nephrectomy: Surgical removal of the kidney.

Nurse anesthetist: A nurse who has had several years of specialized training in the administration of anesthesia.

Nurse practitioner: A nurse with special training who is licensed to diagnose and treat common medical illnesses.

Nursing aide: Health care worker with no specialized training who assists in daily patient care responsibilities.

Nursing assistant: Also known as a nursing aide.

O

Occupational therapist: Health care worker with organized schooling and a degree in helping patients get back to their normal daily living standards after an illness.

Ophthalmologist: Physician who specializes in diseases of the eyes.

Opioids: Class of narcotic drugs that relieve pain.

Oncologist: Physicians specializing in cancer and cancer treatment.

Open Reduction and Internal Fixation (ORIF): Surgical placement of a metal rod or plate to repair bone fractures.

Orthotist: A maker and fitter of orthopaedic appliances.

Otolaryngologist: Physician specializing in diseases of the ear, nose, and throat (ENT).

Otolaryngology: Medical specialty for treating diseases of the ear, nose, and throat.

Otosclerosis: Abnormal formation of new bone around the small bones of the inner ear which can result in deafness.

P

Pancreas: Abdominal organ located behind the stomach, involved in digestion and the control of blood sugar.

Paraplegic: Paralysis below the waist.

Parkinson's Disease: Neurologic disorder of the brain resulting in tremor and rigidity.

Pathologist: Physician trained to examine tissues and organs removed during surgery in order to arrive at a diagnosis.

Patient-Controlled Anesthesia (PCA): Device applied after surgery which allows patients to give themselves narcotic pain medicine when the need arises.

Percutaneous Transluminal Coronary Angioplasty (PTCA): Procedure performed by a cardiologist using a balloon to open up blockages in the main arteries of the heart.

Peripheral nerve stimulator: Device utilizing electric current to stimulate nerves in the body.

Pharmacist: Health care worker with formal schooling in filling prescription medications.

Phlebotomist: Health care worker trained to draw blood from patients in the hospital.

Physical therapist: Health care worker with a formal education and degree in the field of physical therapy who helps patients regain physical strength after surgery or an illness.

Physician's assistant: Health care worker with formal training in caring for patients under the supervision of a physician.

Pneumonia: An infection in the lungs.

Positron Emission Tomography (PET): Highly specialized x-ray imaging using photon technology to detect cancerous tumors.

Post-Anesthesia Care Unit (PACU): Area designated in the hospital where patient are taken immediately after an operation to recover from surgery.

Post-traumatic stress syndrome: Mental illness occurring some time after mental or physical trauma.

Primary surgeon: The surgeon who performs an operation and has primary responsibility for a patient's care.

Primary care physician: Medical doctor, usually a family physician or internist.

Prostate gland: Walnut-shaped gland, located above the bladder in men, which produces semen.

Prostatectomy: Surgical removal of the prostate gland.

Prosthetist: Individual skilled in constructing and fitting prostheses.

Pulmonary: Relating to the lungs.

Pulse oximeter: Machine which continuously measures the level of oxygenation in the blood through a small device attached to a finger tip or ear lobe.

Q

Quadriplegic: Paralysis of muscles and nerves from the neck down.

R

Radiation therapy technologist: Health care worker who assists doctors in the administration of radiation to treat cancer.

Radiologist: Physician trained to perform and interpret x-ray studies taken to arrive at a diagnosis.

Rectum: Lower part of the colon.

Regional anesthesia: Anesthesia which causes a part of the body, such as an arm, a hand, or an ankle, to be numb so a surgeon can perform painless surgery.

Registered nurse (RN): A nurse with a formal degree who has passed a state examination and is licensed to practice nursing.

Renal: Of or relating to the kidneys.

Rhinoplasty: Surgical procedure to reshape the nose.

Residency: Period of physician's training after graduating from medical school.

Respiratory therapist: A health care worker, with formal training in diseases of the lungs, who administers treatments to hospitalized patients for lung ailments.

S

Salivary gland: Gland that secretes saliva, located in the mouth and below the chin.

Salpingo-oophrectomy: Surgical removal of the ovaries and fallopian tubes in women.

Scalpel: Knife used by surgeons during surgery.

Scrub nurse: A nurse who scrubs inside the operating room and hands sterile instruments to surgeons during surgery.

Sinus: An anatomical space, as in the nasal cavity.

Sinus bradycardia: Abnormal slowing of the heart rate.

Spinal cord: Cord of nerve tissue extending from the base of the skull to the tailbone.

Social Worker: Health care worker responsible for discharge and home arrangements for patients ready to be discharged from the hospital.

Speech therapist: A therapist with a formal education and training in helping patients regain normal speech patterns.

Stent: Metal or plastic tube used to hold a blood vessel open.

Strabismus: Disease of the eye muscles, resulting in abnormal vision.

Supraventricular tachycardia: A disease characterized by an abnormally high and irregular heartbeat.

Sympathetic: Part of the nervous system that controls involuntary reflexes and reactions by organs.

T

Thyroid gland: Organ located in the neck that controls body metabolism.

Thyroidectomy: Surgical removal of all or part of the thyroid gland.

Transcutaneous Electric Nerve Stimulation (TENS): A device placed on the skin and used to treat chronic pain by nerve stimulation.

Tubal ligation: Surgical tying of the fallopian tubes to prevent pregnancy in women.

Twilight sedation: Anesthesia in which lighter sedatives are used to induce a lighter sleep state prior to surgery.

U – V

Ultrasound: X-ray test which uses sound waves to evaluate tissues and organs.

Vagina: Birth canal.

Vasectomy: In men, surgical tying of the spermatic cord located in the scrotum to prevent pregnancy.

Vein: Blood vessel that carries unoxygenated blood toward the heart.

Ventilator: A breathing machine or respirator.

W

Warfarin: A medication used to thin the blood.

XYZ

X-ray: A test using small amounts of radioactivity to evaluate tissues, organs, and bones.

Index

About the Author

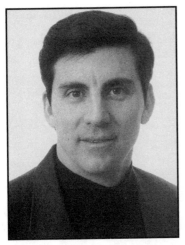

Paul Ruggieri, M.D. is a board-certified general surgeon in private practice in Fall River, Massachusetts. He specializes in thyroid and minimally invasive surgery.

Dr. Ruggieri received his medical degree from the Georgetown University School of Medicine in Washington, D.C. He completed his surgical internship and residency at Barnes Hospital, Washington University School of Medicine, St. Louis, Missouri. After his training, he was stationed at the U.S. Army hospital in Fort Polk, Louisiana. During his time in the military, he rose to the rank of major, received the Army Commendation and Meritorious Service Medals, and became the chief of the department of surgery. In 1995, Dr. Ruggieri entered a private surgical practice near Nashville, Tennessee. In 1998, he returned to his native New England to join a surgical group in southeastern Massachusetts.

Dr. Ruggieri is a fellow in the American College of Surgeons and is a member of the Society of American Gastrointestinal Endoscopic Surgeons.

He is the author of several scientific publications. He is also a contributor to the web site Tradehard.com, where he shares his views on medical technology with the investment community.

Addicus Books
Health & Self-Help Titles

The Family Compatibility Test $9.95
  Susan Adams / 1-886039-27-5

First Impressions—Tips to Enhance Your Image $14.95
  Joni Craighead / 1-886039-26-7

The Healing Touch—Keeping the Doctor/Patient $9.95
  Relationship Alive Under Managed Care
  David Cram, MD / 1-886039-31-3

Hello, Methuselah! Living to 100 and Beyond $14.95
  George Webster, PhD / 1-886039-25-9

Lung Cancer—A Guide to Treatment & Diagnosis $14.95
  Walter J. Scott, MD / 1-886039-43-7 (Spring 2000)

Overcoming Postpartum Depression and Anxiety $12.95
  Linda Sebastian, RN / 1-886930-34-8

Prescription Drug Abuse—The Hidden Epidemic $14.95
  Rod Colvin / 1-886039-22-4

Simple Changes: The Boomer's Guide to a $9.95
  Healthier, Happier Life
  L. Joe Porter, MD / 1-886039-35-6

Straight Talk About Breast Cancer $12.95
  Suzanne Braddock, MD / 1-886039-21-6

The Stroke Recovery Book $14.95
  Kip Burkman, MD / 1-886039-30-5

The Surgery Handbook $14.95
A Guide to Understanding Your Operation
  Paul Ruggieri, MD / 1-886039-38-0

Understanding Parkinson's Disease $14.95
A Self-Help Guide
  David Cram, MD / 1-886039-40-2

Please send:

_____ copies of _____
                                       (Title of book)

at $ _____each   TOTAL   _____

Nebr. residents add 5% sales tax   _____

Shipping/Handling
   $3.20 for first book.
   $1.10 for each additional book.   _____

                TOTAL ENCLOSED: _____

Name_____

Address_____

City _____State _____Zip_____

☐ Visa ☐ Master Card ☐ Am. Express

Credit card number_____Expiration date _____

Order by credit card, personal check or money order. Send to:
Addicus Books
Mail Order Dept.
P.O. Box 45327
Omaha, NE 68145
Or, order **TOLL FREE: 800-352-2873**